PENGUIN BOOKS

SLEEPING LIKE A BABY

Neha Bhatt is an award-winning journalist who reports on public health, human rights, gender and education for leading international and Indian publications. Her work has been published in *The Guardian*, *Al Jazeera*, *The Globe and Mail*, *The British Medical Journal* and *The Hindu*, among others. Formerly a staffer at a range of news organizations, including *Outlook* magazine, she has won the Press Council of India, UNFPA-Laadli and Red Ink awards for excellence in journalism. Neha has also written widely on books, film and culture. She holds a postgraduate diploma from the Asian College of Journalism. She is an advocate for conscious parenting and co-founder of the pioneering support network, Gentle Baby Sleep India. Neha is based in Gurugram, where she lives with her husband and son.

Himani Dalmia is an Australian-Certified Infant and Child Sleep Specialist and co-founder of the support group, Gentle Baby Sleep India. She is a Leader of the La Leche League, the largest non-profit for breastfeeding awareness globally. Her first book, a bestselling and critically acclaimed novel titled *Life Is Perfect*, was published in 2009. Formerly a member of the Times of India Edit Page team, she has contributed widely to newspapers, magazines and journals. A children's picture book by her is currently under publication by HarperCollins India. Himani graduated with honours in English from St. Stephen's College, University of Delhi, and holds a master's degree in South Asian Literature from the University of Oxford. She lives in New Delhi with her husband Akash and two little girls, Devika and Yamini.

ADVANCE PRAISE

'Himani and Neha have written a gem of a book packed with useful information for new and prospective parents. They have thoughtfully applied the concept of biologically normal infant sleep to the concerns of Indian parents having noted in their online parenting community that the discourse regarding where babies' needs arise from was missing from parents' understanding of their babies' sleep patterns and preferences. Their overall approach is very much aligned with the outcomes of our research regarding the importance of encouraging parents to understand and foster biologically normal infant sleep, including nursing to sleep, safe bedsharing, contact napping, experimenting and adapting to meet babies' changing needs, and avoiding sleep training.'

—Helen Ball, Professor of Anthropology, Durham University;
Director, Durham Infancy & Sleep Centre;
Director, Baby Sleep Information Source

'No parenting subject has been more fraught than infant sleep—and none has been as muddied by misinformation and everyday violence. It thrills me that at last we see a book in India that lays bare the myths associated with baby sleep, and leads parents with authority towards a path that is aligned with the biological sleep needs of mum and baby. This book is important for more reasons that I can list—but especially because it is empowering. It grants mothers the permission they so desperately need to hold their babies (well past toddlerhood), share sleep with them on the same bed, tune into the instincts they're otherwise made to suppress, and know the joy and security and restfulness that such an arrangement brings.

Our children don't need sleep training. They need us, their nurturers. They need our warm bodies, the embrace of our willing arms, as they drift into sleep. Himani Dalmia and Neha Bhatt—by deftly weaving together scientific fact and lived experience—remind us of precisely this.'

—Dharini Bhaskar, Mother and Author of
These, Our Bodies, Possessed by Light

'It is so wonderful to see a book on sleep that blends the cross-cultural and historical practices that are covered in-depth in anthropological research with the modern, Western science on sleep. For too long, families have been told they should be pushing independence when it comes to sleep; and yet, what children need in order to feel safe and secure is to be close to a parent. It is unfortunate that Western obsessions regarding sleep—that are not rooted in our human biology—are leaving families exhausted and frustrated. Help that is rooted in ancient traditions that are closely aligned with our biology and psychology is what families need more of, and that is exactly what Neha and Himani can offer tired parents. As a co-sleeping parent myself, I can say the benefits of co-sleeping are not to be underestimated for our sleep but also for our sense of closeness and connection!'

—Tracy Cassels, Founder of Evolutionary Parenting

'This book addresses a core question for every new family - how do we get our baby to sleep? While reading this book I learnt that the question itself was incorrect. Our modern lifestyles end up ruining our children's natural sleep rhythms due to a lack of understanding on our part. As a result, Indian children are some of the most sleep-deprived in the world. This has a massive impact on their daytime emotional regulation and frustration tolerance. Chronically overstimulated children are cranky, prone to tantrums and difficult to feed and soothe. Disrupted sleep cycles are also associated with hyperactivity, inattention and impulsivity – which might help explain the huge rise in these diagnoses in children.

In a gentle, firm, calming voice that impressively even manages to include the political, the authors will hand-hold you toward this understanding of better sleep for everyone at home. I was in tears by the time I had got past the introduction, recalling our struggles as a young family and wishing we had had this book as a guide when we had little babies.'

—Nupur Dhingra Paiva, Clinical Psychologist; Founder and Lead Child & Adolescent Psychotherapist, Family Tree; Author of *Love & Rage: The Inner Worlds of Children*

'When it comes to infant feeding and sleeping arrangements, including scientifically accurate information about infant sleep development and what parents can expect during infancy and beyond, and especially how to foster nighttime safety, comfort and developmental benefits for mothers and infants alike, to my knowledge nobody has done this better than Neha Bhatt and Himani Dalmia in their new book entitled *Sleeping Like a Baby*.'

—James J. McKenna, Dean's Executive Professor, Department of Anthropology, Santa Clara University; Edmund P. Joyce C.S.C Chaired Professor of Anthropology, Emeritus; Director, Mother–Baby Behavioral Sleep Laboratory, Emeritus, University of Notre Dame

'Getting a child to sleep is a big problem for many parents. I would recommend this book to parents who want to understand the art and science of getting this crucial aspect of raising a child right. The book has beautifully covered sleeping patterns, the ways parents can create a conducive environment, practical tips and much more. 237 pages of solid wisdom! Congratulations Neha and Himani for this offering.'

—Anupam Sibal, Paediatric Gastroenterologist; Group Medical Director, Apollo Hospitals; Author of *Is Your Child Ready to Face the World*?

'In the world of thousands of self-help books on babies and sleep, the authors delve into a daunting subject that has deep roots in skewed and biased approaches to sleep. And I must say, *Sleeping Like a Baby* bravely provides a refreshing culture-sensitive, never-before-written book for Indian parents. Neha Bhatt and Himani Dalmia take you right into the heart of ancient wisdom through the lens of challenging modern parenting. The distractions are too many in technologically scattered parenting and living. This book promises to be your companion in this ever secluding world with information on "how best to sleep naturally, biologically, harmoniously".'

—Effath Yasmin, leading International Board Certified Lactation Consultant and Biodynamic Craniosacral Practitioner

SLEEPING LIKE A BABY

The Art and Science
of Gentle Baby Sleep

NEHA BHATT AND **HIMANI DALMIA**

Foreword by

JAMES J. MCKENNA, PHD,
FOUNDER, MOTHER–BABY BEHAVIORAL
SLEEP LABORATORY

PENGUIN BOOKS

An imprint of Penguin Random House

PENGUIN BOOKS

USA | Canada | UK | Ireland | Australia
New Zealand | India | South Africa | China

Penguin Books is part of the Penguin Random House group of companies
whose addresses can be found at global.penguinrandomhouse.com

Published by Penguin Random House India Pvt. Ltd
4th Floor, Capital Tower 1, MG Road,
Gurugram 122 002, Haryana, India

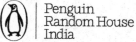

First published in Penguin Books by Penguin Random House India 2021

ISBN 9780143452461

Typeset in Adobe Garamond Pro by Manipal Technologies Limited, Manipal

www.penguin.co.in

For our children
Sahir, Devika and Yamini
for filling our hearts and fitting together
the pieces of the biggest parenting puzzles

Contents

Foreword

'If you are for the right thing, you do it without thinking'

In Maya Angelou's award-winning autobiography, *I Know Why the Caged Bird Sings*, having fallen asleep in bed with her newborn son, Maya expressed relief to her mother upon awakening to find that she hadn't suffocated him as she feared. Her mother reassured her by telling her to have no fears because . . . 'If you are for the right thing, you do it without thinking.'

When it comes to infant feeding and sleeping arrangements, including scientifically accurate information about infant sleep development and what parents can expect during infancy and beyond, and especially how to foster nighttime safety, comfort and developmental benefits for mothers and infants alike, to my knowledge nobody has done this better than Neha Bhatt and Himani Dalmia in their new book entitled *Sleeping Like a Baby*. This remarkably thorough, well-written and evidence-based book represents an impressive *holistic* understanding of *who the human infant is biologically*, the only criteria from which the most optimal recommendations discussed herein can be based, but seldom are, especially in books about infant sleep.

Throughout their book the authors update and correct fallacious imported Western notions about what *truly* constitutes normal, healthy *human* infant sleep development, thereby protecting India's exemplary emphasis on its cherished traditions of breastfeeding while mothers sleep next to their babies—what we call breastsleeping (McKenna and Gettler 2016a). It is this information that provides ample scientific ammunition for refutation when needed against sleep-training advocates, who are supported by associated false social myths, which, as the authors describe, are 'inching closer to our neighbourhoods and parenting circles'.

The integration of insights and knowledge is offered from their own mothering and impressive professional experiences, including interviews (with quotes from mothers themselves), all affirmed by the best scientific research; it certainly reads as a breath of fresh air. Every step of the way the book empowers and reassures mothers who, even in India, sometimes find resistance and/or warnings against sleeping with their babies. Such a fallacious *Euro-American perspective* dismisses and/or fails to acknowledge the importance of breastsleeping, a complex, interdependent set of behaviours that induce uniquely human physiological and neurobiological processes, representing an evolved, highly successful human adaptation hundreds of thousands of years old. It represents a critical, singular bio-cultural system that offers a credible explanation for how one primate mammal, the human infant, could possibly survive such a prolonged period of neuro-biological dependence and immaturity, especially when born with only 25 per cent of its adult brain volume. That is only made possible by the co-evolution of a cooperation-based, intense and prolonged degree of parental investment, including intense contact, carrying and 'sleeping with babies' (McKenna 2018, McKenna and Gettler 2016a, McKenna and Gettler 2016b).

Let me note that in the USA many sleep-training clinics are popping up, using aggressive unfounded tactics put forth in advertisements by ill-trained 'experts'. It still surprises me how convincing these persons can be. One explanation is that these 'experts' use their words and their educational degrees as weapons to scare parents while dismissing the importance of mothers' own acquired knowledge, their experiences and feelings, and their overall abilities as mothers to come to know just what their infants need, perhaps better than anyone else.

And what is that which is learned? Indeed, universally and regardless of what culture each infant is born into, mothers and fathers everywhere are quick to learn that in addition to breastmilk infants need contact, contact, and more contact. As anthropologist Ashley Montagu argued decades ago, this is because the human neonate-infant is born as an 'extero-gestate', and finishes its gestation after birth, during what others call the 'fourth trimester'. Montagu went on to say that universally, all human infants are 'contact seekers' as the neonate's genes at this stage are close to the surface, having control over the infant's behaviours. Contact seeking is instinctual among infants and takes the form of an irrepressible reflex that will not and cannot be nullified by recent cultural changes that argue to minimize nighttime contact with infants for fear of 'spoiling them', or creating a 'bad habit' or a 'clingy' baby. But these tenacious old-fashioned notions, as the book makes apparent, have literally nothing to do with infants at all, and everything to do with recent social ideologies and speculations. These begin by defining infants *not* in terms of who they are biologically, as mentioned above, but in terms of someone's version of what *they* want infants to become, and their incorrect notions about how to get infants to be of that 'right' personality, i.e., independent, which is to make the infant sleep alone, ostensibly (but not really) signifying the infants 'independence', all by four months of age! (McKenna and Gettler 2016b). Thankfully, many scholars in this field, myself included, see infant sleep training as cruel, victimizing babies for being babies; nonetheless it represents a position that advocates claim has science behind it. It doesn't, as Neha and Himani make known emphatically! I love it and I agree whole heartedly when they say: 'We believe independence comes in its own time as children grow, *even if you do nothing to hurry it along*. Forcing independence on children leads to major behavioural issues later.'

The point is that one of the unique features of this book is the diversity of vibrant and current examples, and the many lines of scientific evidence that shows that there is no such thing as giving an infant too much attention and, hence, being overly 'indulgent'. This reminds me of the 'father' of American psychology, David Watson, and his famous contradicting quote. He said, 'It is not possible to give infants too little attention'. No wonder America got off on such a wrong track when it comes to what is, in fact, healthy sleep and sleeping arrangements for the infant. Unfortunately, Watson serving as a powerful influence on past thinking about healthy infant and childhood behaviours was helped along by three other white middle-aged men with medical degrees. Two of them wrote bestselling care books: Emmett Holt and Benjamin Spock. Sigmund Freud dominated psychiatric circles with his Electra and Oedipus theories, which sexualized infants and parental psychoses, certainly nailing the coffin shut regarding any possibility that sleeping with one's baby would be thought of as normal and/or appropriate. Sadly, they wrote their recommendations without any of them ever changing a diaper nor ever using empirical or actual observational or biological studies of infants as the basis for their recommendations. All of their pronouncements were based on social values and cultural ideologies and/or perceptions of potential infant–adult psychoses. The bottom line is they all strongly recommended that shortly after birth, as soon as possible, babies should sleep alone.

But, many years later, the return of breastfeeding to Western industrialized societies changed everything. Indeed, despite attempts to eradicate bedsharing in the USA by the American Academy of Pediatrics, the rates of bedsharing are increasing. Through behaviours such as baby-led breastfeeding, cuddling, carrying, baby wearing, holding (all discussed in the book), it becomes clear why sleeping with one's baby is not just a nice social idea, as is being made explicit by more evolution-based, contemporary, empirical infancy research (see Ball et al. 2020 for a review). Rather, these proximity-maintaining activities necessarily function positively within and outside of the breastfeeding dyad. Moreover, the biological functional connections between breastfeeding and co-sleeping, especially, are so powerful and interdependent that my colleague, Dr Lee Gettler, and I took the opportunity to create a new word for it—breastsleeping—about which Neha and Himani also speak (see McKenna and Gettler 2016a).

But to elaborate a bit, it must be understood that maternal infant contact functions to regulate and compensate for the human infant's extreme neurological immaturity at birth, which explains how and why sustained parent–infant contact day or night asserts physiological regulatory effects. These are, for example, influencing heartbeat intervals, blood pressure, stress levels (mediated by the cortisol and oxytocin production), sleep–wake patterns, including sleep stage duration and sleep cycle (stage length), infant body temperature, body orientations and positions during breastsleeping in bed, infant oxygenations, breathing patterns including apnea durations and distribution across infant sleep stages, arousal patterns, and breastfeeding frequency and duration over time. Increased parental contact also positively influences digestive efficiency (growth rate itself) as American psycho-biologist Tiffany Field demonstrated decades ago. More recent data shows how increased breastmilk ingestion helps by way of oligosaccharides, which feed 'good bacteria' in the infant's gut needed for the infant's healthy microbiome, in addition to providing hundreds of home-grown antibodies, proteins, enzymes, minerals, fatty acids and stem cells that place the developmental trajectory of the infant's immune system especially in the direction of both short- and long-term health (Ball et al. 2020, McKenna et al. 2007, Blair et al. 2020). Neha and Himani clearly generically discuss these regulatory effects using multiple lines of evidence that show how and why the 'Indian approach' to nighttime infant sleep and feeding practices represents a biologically appropriate micro-environment for the human infant, particularly in sustaining overall optimal development.

In the West, although things are beginning to change with something like one to two million new mothers breastsleeping and for longer periods, still, the literature surrounding these issues often conceptualize forms of co-sleeping but especially bedsharing as inherently dangerous (except for separate surface roomsharing, which is supported). Moreover, infants themselves are often portrayed as potential adversaries of the mother or father primed to induce parents to *do their bidding* (so-to-speak) and, hence, sleep training, however cruel and unnecessary, can seem like a logical and necessary parental defense and intervention.

But this cultural meme that infants have agendas, or that they 'want' something, which involves cognition (which they do not yet have), is ludicrous. Infants for at least 4 to 6 months have no 'wants' but only 'needs', because at this point the human infant's genes are finding direct expression with a human infant lacking any ability to control his or her feelings, or to display behavioural strategies such as 'manipulating' their mothers and fathers. Indian parents, from my distant view, seem to understand this.

I should also add that the comprehensiveness with which Neha and Himani put forth critical corrections to the Euro-American infant sleep mythologies (presently knocking at India's cultural borders) is unique insofar as they include what parents should expect not just with regard to infant sleep but how toddlers' and children's sleep patterns change and progress over time—not usually in a linear manner, especially in the first year of life but also throughout the first five years. Few infant sleep books I know of take the parents on such an expanded, age-specific, informative journey, which no doubt will be greatly appreciated by parents.

Finally, what comes across loud and clear in *Sleeping Like a Baby* is the reality that the decisions parents make as to what their caregiving practices expose infants to in terms of social which is simultaneously physical if not intellectual (as sensory maternal-infant engagements are now known to play a critical role in the parents' ability to influence the direction and quality of brain growth including degrees of inter-neuronal connectivity and neuronal density), lay down a kind of neurological scaffolding and trajectory for both present and future levels of infant cognition and intellectual expansion. For example, information eluded to in this book is reflective of recent magnetic resonation studies of infant brain development that reveal the potential ways enriched early sensory and social engagements of infants with their parents and others can retain young neurons that would otherwise be permanently lost. What babies are exposed to environmentally likely changes the migration of immature neurons that start off on a journey to the prefrontal cortex on the first day of post-natal life, starting as a mass of young undeveloped 'peri neurons' hiding behind the infant's eyes, which were not known to exist until just five or so years ago (see Paredes et al. 2016). What is even more amazing is that as they journey, it is very likely that based on what the infant is socially and physically experiencing (this is my inference) these undeveloped *peri* neurons mature into functionally different neuron 'types' (a fact discovered by Paredes et al. 2016). And where exactly these neurons end up in the prefrontal cortex could likewise be dependent on, or influenced by, the caregiving choices made by the infant's parents (again, my inference or proposal).

This migration of neurons to the prefrontal cortex located in and around the forehead region is what is called the 'seat of executive functioning', the location in the brain where judgement, evaluation, purposeful behaviour, reasoning, stop-go activities, decision-making and even potentially mental health resiliency originates (see Parades et al. 2016). This adds to the overall positive effects of increased maternal–infant contact with breastfeeding. Likewise, Deoni et al. (2013) found that exclusively breastfeeding babies compared with non-breastfeeding babies develop a significantly higher density of white matter (glial cell neurons) responsible for fast messaging and inter-neuronal communication up and down the spinal cord, essentially integrating the entire nervous system into a singular system. These studies surely suggest emphatically that parents can inadvertently play a more essential role in influencing the kind of brain their children will grow.

All the scientific, creative, thoughtful, and mother-inspired knowledge leading to situationally sensitive recommendations brought together in this marvellous book certainly answers an abundance of sleep and related developmental questions, not the least of which are why bedsharing and breastsleeping are safe and beneficial for babies, and why it is worth protecting. Perhaps authors Neha Bhatt and Himani Dalmia as well as Maya Angelou's mother will not mind me reminding us all once again that, as regards breastsleeping and other forms of safe co-sleeping, 'when you are for the right thing, you do it without thinking'. Surely, 'sleeping with baby' is the 'right thing', but also is reading this book, which will help parents to know exactly what they need to know as they make informed decisions regarding their infant's and/or child's more optimal care and well being.

James J. McKenna, PhD, Dean's Executive Professor, Department of Anthropology, Santa Clara University; Edmund P. Joyce C.S.C Chaired Professor of Anthropology, Emeritus; and Director, Mother–Baby Behavioral Sleep Laboratory, Emeritus, University of Notre Dame

Introduction

There are two kinds of people in this world: those who sleep well and those who don't. In modern life, alarmingly, more and more adults and children fall into the latter category. A sign of our times, perhaps? But it could also be our lack of understanding of what it takes to sleep. From morning to night, through our chaotic days, there is an overwhelming number of barriers to sleep. We are almost constantly caught in the web of busy schedules, flooded with artificial light, multiple screens scrambling for our attention, bogged down by stress and anxiety.

But it's only when you become a parent that the lack of sleep pushes you to the brink and makes you rethink a lot of choices you make daily. A few weeks into parenthood, you realize no one told you how to fix this problem when you were preparing to welcome a child into your home.

Sleep deprivation is an inherent part of early parenthood. But it doesn't have to be a constant part of parenthood. This is why we decided to write this book—we found there are a great deal of myths to dispel and expectations to bust and a huge awareness gap to fill in Indian society.

Look around you: How many parents do you know who struggle with their children's sleep? How many believe their children do not like to sleep? Chances are you know more than a handful. The truth is it doesn't have to be this way. You *can* find a way out of sleep deprivation and reset your expectations from your child and, most of all, from yourself.

How It Began

Indian children are among the most sleep-deprived in the world: they barely clock 8 hours of sleep a night instead of the prescribed 10–12 hours, besides naps for younger children. Why do Indian parents struggle to get their children to bed? Why are Indian children among the most sleep-deprived in the world?

When we became parents, a year apart, we were almost instantly drawn to this mystery that seemed to puzzle most Indian families. Our children, meanwhile, seemed to quickly fall into healthy, age-appropriate sleep routines, as we applied a mix of ancient wisdom and new-age research to manage their sleep. Having known each other from school, we reconnected when we realized that we share a common passion for baby sleep.

As we dug into the research, we decided to probe some of the burning sleep-related questions of the day: are babies really 'poor sleepers' as millions of parents believe? In our common parenting networks, online and offline, we began to ask new mothers and fathers a series of questions to understand the underlying problems. Many began to seek our advice on hearing our personal stories of success with baby sleep. We were happy to share our formulae, backed by international research, globally accepted sleep guidelines and the intricate and well-documented science behind child sleep and its links to growth and development.

Alarmed at the scale of sleep deprivation across families, we found that India has a serious sleep crisis that runs deep, across most homes. It does not help that there is a severe lack of India-based research and basic awareness on the importance of children having an age-appropriate sleep routine. There had to be a way to bridge this gap. And thus, Gentle Baby Sleep India (GBSI), a support network on Facebook for new parents, was born. We founded this group in February 2016, intending to foster gentle, no-cry methods to inculcate healthy sleep habits in babies and toddlers.

Within a few months, we found thousands of parents flocking to our group. At the time of writing this book, we have more than 50,000 members, with hundreds of joining requests daily, more than our 10-member voluntary admin team can handle.

Along the way, Himani became accredited as a Leader of the La Leche League, the largest breastfeeding support non-profit globally, and began to offer voluntary mother-to-mother support on lactation as well. Soon after, she became certified by the Institute of Sensitive Sleep in Australia as a baby sleep counsellor, after a rigorous, research-based course. In addition to her voluntary work on GBSI, she provides professional, one-to-one support to parents as well. This involves a long-term association with families where their baby's sleep is tracked over weeks and months. Her formal training and intensive relationship with parents has given Himani a breadth of knowledge and deep insight on baby sleep, brought into sharp focus by her years of experience on GBSI. Neha, meanwhile, a longtime journalist who covers public health, social justice and gender issues, devoted her free time to co-lead and mentor the GBSI team and worked voluntarily as a baby sleep guide to parents on GBSI. She is also a conscious parenting advocate.

And now, dear reader, we have put it all down for you in this book. It's designed to be your go-to sleep bible, your bedside companion as you take baby steps into the art of parenting.

What You Will Find in This Book

A few months ago, we conducted a sleep survey on 'Sleep Patterns in Children and Parental Response' that studied observations of nearly 800 parents. The results were telling. Over 40 per cent reported they didn't know anything about baby sleep before joining GBSI. Their chief concerns were that their child is awake most of the day, sleeps very late at night and resists sleep. Others struggled with their baby needing artificial sleep aids such as cradles, swings, pacifiers and bottles to sleep.

Most parents who join our group put out an urgent plea for help: 'My baby won't sleep! What should I do?' Worryingly, many express feelings of intense anxiety, depression and exhaustion because they are confused about why their baby doesn't sleep the way they want him/her to. What compounds the issue is receiving conflicting bits of advice from friends and family (such as 'keep your baby awake during the day so that she sleeps at night', 'don't let your baby fall asleep in your arms', or 'feed your baby formula or solids so that he sleeps longer hours') that tend to be at odds with a child's biological needs. In our group, with the help of the resources we have put together along with personalized, need-based advice, most babies fall into age-appropriate routines and parents are reassured that they are not, after all, bad parents with children who are poor sleepers. The advice we offer, which is tweaked now and then to suit every parent's specific situation, is designed to equip caregivers with enough knowledge to ride the choppy waters of baby sleep like experienced sailors.

Our mission, though, goes deeper to challenge systemic issues. The immense sleep deprivation that comes with early parenthood has given rise to a massive sleep training industry in the West, and the publication of hundreds of books on baby sleep. While there is certainly an eager audience for sleep books the world over, there is no Indian book on the subject, marrying our cultural practices with the best that modern science has to offer. Our 'secret' is not to be found in any sleep book we have encountered from any part of the world. Yet, this same formula can be applied to any baby in the world, with guaranteed results. What we do night and day is to bring your baby closer to you, bridging a divide that parents tend to feel when it's bedtime. On those occasions, when you despair and wonder what's going on, you might find the answer in this book. (Don't wait for that moment though—we recommend reading *Sleeping Like a Baby* before things get out of hand!)

Five years after we started GBSI, we have hundreds of success stories we feel proud of. When members write 'gratitude posts' telling us how the recommendations changed their days for the better and fostered a deeper connection with their baby, we feel that our job is done. Many members tell us how the group has helped them bridge intergenerational divides too, with grandparents equally convinced about following age-appropriate routines after seeing the results. When we asked parents in our survey how much the group's recommendations (of sleep schedules, awake windows, avoiding overtiredness, bridging naps, dark and quiet rooms, holding for naps, nursing to sleep and bedsharing) helped them in their baby sleep journey, the answers were heartening. Over 45 per cent reported moderate improvement, 37 per cent said they found major improvement with steady, consistent implementation over months and 9 per cent said they found dramatic improvement within a few days.

As we thought about the wealth of personal experiences and data on baby and toddler sleep (0–5 years) we have gathered over the years, we realized that to do justice to this vast and intriguing subject, we had to put it all down in a concrete form that would hopefully help new parents beyond the group.

In here, you will find deeply researched, first-hand accounts on understanding sleep cycles, how to manage baby sleep regressions, breastfeeding and sleep, baby sleep for working parents, how to make sure kids get enough sleep once they start school, how to inculcate a bedtime reading habit, managing sleep in the context of the joint Indian family and much more.

Our goal in writing *Sleeping Like a Baby* was to put together an instructive and exhaustive handbook that blends research with anecdotes, which draws on traditional wisdom as well as nuances of modern parenting. Between these pages, you will explore case studies of mothers and fathers like you and us who struggled with sleep and overcame their issues, and you will read perspectives from well-known international sleep experts, doctors and researchers who have studied sleep in children in ancient and modern life.

So, as we set out to decode the many mysteries of how young children sleep, we equally wanted to make the point that sleep is not always about the maths of routines and schedules, and the science of sleep. It is deeply linked to your style of parenting and the connections that form between you and your children from even before the time they are born. It is one of the reasons we recommend that parents read this book when they are pregnant or very early on in their parenting journey. It's 100 per cent true that the more you bond with your child, the easier it is to build healthy sleep habits. Without a respectful, loving, attached relationship, it is very hard to follow the path of gentle sleep and indeed even ensure good sleep for the whole family. You could have the best routine in the world, the most excellent sleep environment and yet your child will struggle with sleep if there is something amiss in your relationship and in your home. You will notice that even your daily anxieties and stress will affect your child's sleep. As we often tell parents, if you find that your baby or toddler is struggling to sleep despite all the parameters being snugly in place, check if there is something troubling you, your immediate family environment and if it is in any way affecting your connection with your children. If that is indeed the case, we suggest seeking whatever help you need to plug those gaps while also examining your parenting style and digging deeper into your own anxieties and fears. Parenting has a way of showing you the mirror, and sometimes what looks back at you is not what you want to see. Children tend to pick up on our worst habits and fears. When you become a parent, you travel back to your childhood and see it through a different lens. Along the way, you learn to deal with some of the wounds you carry with you and this can help immensely in deepening your link to your child and the ways in which your lives are intertwined. And connection is everything, especially when it comes to sleep. If you expect your toddler to march off to bed the moment you tell her it is bedtime, your expectations are askew. It is pointless to expect robotic behaviour from children, because they need security, love and connection while sleeping (and while doing everything else) just as much as adults.

The Feminist Politics of Baby Sleep

As pro-choice feminists, we have often been baffled by the suggestion that, to be a good feminist, you absolutely must put your own needs before your child's. We often hear that for women who leave the home to work, children's needs are inconvenient and must be clipped in order to serve a larger feminist purpose. There is also the suggestion that stay-at-home parents can deal better with night wakings than parents who have to step out to do paid work. In our collective experience of having done it all at different points—stepping out to an office to work, working from home, taking time off paid work—we found that children's biological impulses remain the same, no matter your career choices. Though the larger gender debate on the unfair burden of caregiving on women has demanded the male parent step up, in practice, the onus often falls on children to realign their needs and the co-parent simply does not go the distance. At any given point in time during the first five years of your child's life, shifting priorities by both parents has a magical effect on your child's well being. What those shifting priorities look like, which we discuss in detail in this book, is a decision that must be taken by every parent and every family in the way that works best for them, but children's basic rights should be kept in mind. We believe that being aware and respectful of a child's developmental needs is important and not inferior to our career concerns. Parenting is never a one-track journey and phases come and go. By investing time and energy in the first few years—again, by both parents or multiple caregivers—into your baby's sleep does not translate to you giving up your whole life to raise children. Children, whether you like it or not, do become hugely independent on their own, allowing your career to organically become stronger, deeper and more fulfilling as they grow.

There is a historical context to our argument. The idea of feeding infant formula as a regular practice and sleep training gained traction during the women's liberation movement of the 1970s. Increasingly, there has been a philosophy in the decades that followed that women need to fulfill their professional destinies, be financially independent, and not be shackled to home and hearth. While this has led to a fair amount of social justice and progress for women, things have come almost full circle on motherhood in particular. Women born into a relatively freer world have, in fact, felt the oppression of the pressure to 'have it all'. With increasing research on the harmful effects of sleep training and the benefits of following biological norms, mothers (and indeed fathers) have tuned into their biological instincts and found it to be at odds with what society is asking them to do with their babies. Sleep training, early weaning from the breast, early separation into institutionalized childcare, negative discipline aimed at fostering early and unnatural independence have begun to feel dissonant to many parents. In this scenario, parents who choose to follow the biologically normal approach, which may include one or both parents prioritizing childcare over careers, often face censure over their seemingly 'anti-feminist' choices. The fact is, the way in which social and economic structures currently exist make it difficult for parents to meet the biological needs of their infants. Extended paternity and maternity leave, flexible work arrangements, creches within offices, increased normalization of breastfeeding in public, easier options for mums or dads to return to work after a break would support parents to provide the kind of hands-on, connection-based care that young babies really need. Even so, a mother following her instincts and choosing to nurture a baby for a while before returning to the workforce is in fact exercising a choice. Making choices intricately linked to a woman's body in a world built by men is never easy. We hope that this book will provide tools, strategies, support and even permission to women who wish to embrace baby-led parenting.

Whose Right Is It Anyway?

Another burning issue that we address in this book is the complex subject of childism. Childism is essentially holding prejudice against children, treating them like we own them and like they must be told what to do, while disrespecting their needs, choices and natural instincts. It can be as simple as dismissing a baby's request to be held or forcing a child to eat when she makes it clear she is not hungry. Cumulatively, when we think about how much we hold against children across the world—that they are manipulative, they demand too much attention, they are needy and clingy and need to be scolded or spanked to instil discipline, and so on and so forth—we find that it is an entire culture built to think the worst of them. Truthfully, children come into the world absolutely perfectly equipped with all the tools they need to grow. It's all pretty much in-built and will sprout at the age it is meant to, given the right conditions and care. They need our support, guidance and deep attachment and security. It's their right to lead the way, to give us cues on what they need and how they feel. Setting boundaries for their safety and helping them understand right from wrong is our job too; however, this can be done in a respectful way without trampling on their feelings so that the relationship and growth is a collaboration rather than a power struggle, which parenting too often curdles into. Childism is no less offensive and problematic than sexism, racism and outright child abuse. The difference is that childism, slightly more general in nature, can be almost impossible to identify for most parents because it is so ingrained in how we interact not just with our own children but children in general. Not many know it exists. But becoming aware is the first step to rearranging the power equation between our children and all of us, the adults around them, in a way that they do not feel subjugated and treated as lesser than grown people. How is this connected to sleep? Sleep is not an isolated activity; it ties in with everything we do and experience during the day. So, as we argue in this book, in order to align your child's sleep habits with biological needs, we need to, at every point, advocate for our children. In many places in the book, you will find that we try to speak for your children. This is because parenting can frequently be so overwhelming that often our own needs as adults are not met, and when we are hurting and stressed out and feeling frustrated with the clash between reality and expectations, it is hard to see things from the point of view of your children. We have been there too. Seeing it from a distance now, we want to do our bit to restore that balance in your home, if we can.

What You Won't Find in This Book

If there's one thing we do not stand for, it is 'sleep training'. Through this book, we challenge the idea that children need to be sleep-trained by letting them cry or causing them discomfort, as is commonly believed by sleep consultants in the West and now increasingly in India. Instead, we hope this book will empower parents to trust their child's basic instincts and guide them to establish healthy sleep habits in a gentle and humane way that can last a lifetime and completely turn the way people look at parenting.

We will not tell you in this book that you must get your baby used to self-soothing. We will not tell you to wean your baby early from the breast to enable self-soothing. We will not explain how to make your baby a more independent sleeper. We believe independence comes in its own time as children grow, even if you do nothing to hurry it along. Forcing independence on children leads to major behavioural issues later. We will not tell you to move your children to a separate room or a separate sleeping surface to 'make them sleep better'.

In short, we will not tell you to do anything that jeopardizes the parent–child bond in any way. Our goal is to facilitate a gentle and loving relationship between parents and children through the realm of sleep based on empathy and science. We would like to help parents view baby sleep from the perspective of their children, who are too young to articulate how they feel. We are here to listen to you, new parents, but more than that, we are here for your babies. The person who will benefit most from this book is your baby because the emotional, physiological and mental welfare of your baby is our highest priority.

A Warning

The information in this book can sound quite revolutionary at first (and hence the need to write this book). The fact that it can seem so different from what your peers and elders have advised and what Google searches throw up through search-engine-optimized sleep training sites can come as a shock. The realization that you've been doing things wrong can be potentially upsetting. Despair not! Help is here. This is the advice that, when implemented, will feel right.

Why 'Sleeping Like a Baby'?

The term 'sleeping like a baby' is misunderstood and misused to refer to someone who 'sleeps like a log'. We would like to reclaim the phrase because, ironically, babies do not sleep simply or deeply but in their distinct ways, and there are ways for parents to embrace this. We know that age-appropriate sleep is the secret to happy, well-adjusted children who rarely throw tantrums, rarely feel cranky and do well both at home and at school. They eat better, imbibe better than peers who are sleep-deprived and can manage their emotions like little champs.

So, on that warm note, dear reader, welcome aboard.

Notes: Some names have been changed to protect the identities of the case study subjects.

The guidelines within this book are based on years of experience of all the GBSI admins put together that have roots in scientific evidence. Though we strongly believe in evidence-based research, the fact is that research on baby sleep that isn't skewed by sleep training bias is quite scant. Hence, we have included references wherever possible, but the methods have been refined and enhanced by the collective experience of over 20 admins with more than 30 babies between them and years of practical experience advising thousands of parents, providing hands-on support and tweaking on a real-time basis. Along the way, we have learnt what works for different families and what doesn't, so, we have offered variations of each method. If issues persist which you believe (or suspect) are medical, please speak to a certified healthcare professional. We do not advise on medical issues.

The terms 'he' and 'she' are used interchangeably for babies. The terms 'mother/father/parent' refer, in most cases, to all primary caregivers. The term 'father', in particular, denotes any non-breastfeeding co-parent in any type of family.

1

Sleep in Ancient Cultures

If there's one thing we can say with certainty about the history of sleep, it's that our ancestors didn't sleep like we do today.

So, how did they sleep? We are beginning to find some answers, studying modern hunter–gatherer cultures to gain some insight into how our early ancestors slept.

As a civilization, we're at a crossroads. Across the world, we're digging deep into the biological factors that make us who we are, why we behave the way we do, the basic instincts that make up our framework and provide answers to essential questions about Homo sapiens. In this exploration, scientists and researchers are finding that the mysterious trail back to our origins is peppered with traditional wisdom.

Studies of cultural practices that our ancestors followed have revealed an instinctive approach to everything for survival. In modern times, however, this wisdom that came to us biologically, like an impulse, has been forced to retreat to the shadows for the sake of convenience as we have forged a path to economic growth. Along the way, we have dispensed with some of those impulses that have protected us for centuries.

Experts are now pausing to reflect on what we've left behind. Even as we chant the various mantras of good living—'eat what your grandmother ate', 'grow your own food', 'slow down', 'listen to your body', 'ditch the artificial for the natural', etc.—let's understand how best to sleep naturally, biologically, harmoniously. To do that, let's go back to the beginning, to when humans slept in the wild.

How They Slept

In 2014, an experiment to investigate how people slept in prehistoric living conditions proved insightful. The researchers found that in the absence of modern living conditions—such as screens and artificial light, and stressful, busy routines—the subjects of the study went to sleep earlier and slept longer. These are the conditions that children too sleep best in.

More importantly, as several other findings have shown, early tribes shared common sleeping space, children attached to their parents, and families wrapped up work by sunset and woke up at sunrise. Leaving babies in separate spaces, away from their caregivers, day or night, was simply not a consideration. Babies fed and slept according to their biological needs and thrived when attached firmly to their caregivers. Those who weren't, didn't survive, and were eaten up by wild animals.

Bestselling author and paediatrician Carlos González in the excellent parenting bible *Kiss Me: How to Raise Your Children with Love* writes,

> Mothers who left their children alone for more than a few
> minutes soon had no children. Their genes were eliminated
> by natural selection. By contrast, the genes that compelled

mothers to stay with their children were passed down to numerous descendants. You are one of those descendants. Modern women have a natural genetic inclination to stay with their children . . .

In the book, González explains the simple truth behind why children sleep better when they are close to their caregivers and why they resist sleeping alone.

A series of studies led by Darcia Narvaez, professor of Psychology at the University of Notre Dame, went a step further to examine the effects of such an arrangement. It was concluded that child-rearing practices in foraging hunter–gatherer societies—like holding, sleeping close to adult caregivers, responding to children every time they cried and so on—led to 'better mental health, greater empathy and conscience development, and higher intelligence in children'. In modern societies, she found, 'an increased level of aggression, anxiety and depression is linked with depriving children of empathy and compassion in the early years'.

In modern life, parents are under tremendous pressure to teach their children to become less dependent on them and sleep independently, without needing a feed from the breast and without physical closeness. In ancient times, this wasn't a logical expectation at all because it was deeply linked to survival. So, you might be correct to think that we are putting unrealistic expectations on ourselves and our children when we expect them to sleep on their own, on a separate sleeping surface such as a cot, before they can utter their first word and fend for themselves in most other ways.

The truth is, our ancestors knew exactly how to sleep. It wasn't considered something anyone had to 'learn'. Babies know how to sleep right from the time they are in the womb, where they sleep 80–90 per cent of the time. In there, they have all the right conditions for a cosy sleep—a warm, dark space to nestle in where they instinctively feel safe and secure, their mother and father's muffled voices drifting in and out of their consciousness, music and lyrics to their ears.

So, when babies come out into the world, wailing and red-faced, they expect the same conditions, which can be somewhat replicated in the warm safety of their parents' arms, while suckling on-demand at the mother's breast and while snoozing softly on a loving caregiver's lap. As González writes in *Kiss Me*:

> The greater the divide between the way we want our children to sleep and the way that comes naturally to them, the more we will need to teach them how to sleep. It is much easier to teach them to sleep in pyjamas or in a bed than it is to teach them to sleep without their mother.

So, you see, when many parents wonder why children don't like being left alone, especially when they're drifting to sleep, the answer lies in the history of humankind and how we are essentially wired.

Our basic instincts are built to crave physical closeness and community life. This is why babies cry when they are left alone—they fear for their lives. Many parents misunderstand crying to be a sign of manipulation. But babies are not capable of manipulation. They are not trying to make life difficult for you. They are only trying to survive, and crying is the only way they know to get your attention to express to you something they don't yet quite have the words for. When they cry, it's to express that they are insecure, or hungry, or need a nappy change. By all accounts, they just need your attention.

During our engagements with the parenting community over the years, we found that it is this anthropological discourse—to understand where babies' needs arise from—that is missing. It is particularly lacking in medical professionals who work with children, such as paediatricians, who are often not well-versed in gentle parenting methods and the biological impulses of babies. There are, of course, exceptions, and we have also encountered the odd paediatrician who recommends natural parenting methods and age-appropriate sleep. But it's rare. The paediatric community's recommendations, particularly in Western cultures, is that children should be trained to sleep separately and should be weaned from night feeds at 6–9 months old. It is now being widely countered by leading experts across the world. One of them is Dr James McKenna, recognized as a leading authority on the subject of mother–infant co-sleeping in relation to breastfeeding and sudden infant death syndrome (SIDS). In his groundbreaking Mother–Baby Behavioral Sleep Laboratory, at the University of Notre Dame, Indiana, he studied through an anthropological lens how sleeping environments reflect and respond to family needs—in particular, how they affect mothers, breastfeeding and infants' physiological and psychological well-being and development. In his paper, 'Mother-Infant Cosleeping with Breastfeeding in the Western Industrialized Context: A Bio-Cultural Perspective', he observes:

> First, be aware that only in the last century have humans anywhere asked where their babies should or would sleep. It is a very 'modern' question not asked by the majority of contemporary people. Indeed, perhaps it is more pertinent

to ask whether billions of people could be wrong? The overwhelming majority of contemporary parents outside the western industrialized world appreciate and accept without question the benefits and necessity, if not the inevitability, of mothers sleeping next to their infants (cosleeping), which is seen as natural and expected, if not morally appropriate.

It is expected that a caregiver will be sleeping next to an infant because babies can't (no one can, really) sleep deeply and restoratively till they feel secure and comforted. This is why the moment you pick your baby up, he/she feels taken care of, and after being nursed or rocked or walked and held close to you, drops right off to sleep. In his paper 'Cosleeping and Biological Imperatives: Why Human Babies Do Not and Should Not Sleep Alone', McKenna argues,

> One of the most important reasons why bedsharing occurs, and the reason why simple declarations against it will not eradicate it, is because sleeping next to one's baby is biologically appropriate, unlike placing infants prone to sleep or putting an infant in a room to sleep by itself. This is particularly so when bedsharing is associated with breast feeding . . . For breastfeeding mothers, bedsharing makes breastfeeding much easier to manage and practically doubles the amount of breastfeeding sessions while permitting both mothers and infants to spend more time asleep. The increased exposure to mother's antibodies which comes with more frequent nighttime breastfeeding can potentially, per any given infant, reduce infant illness. And because co-sleeping in the form of bedsharing makes breastfeeding easier for mothers, it encourages them to breastfeed for a greater

number of months, according to Dr Helen Ball's studies at the University of Durham, therein potentially reducing the mother's chances of breast cancer. Indeed, the benefits of cosleeping helps explain why simply telling parents never to sleep with baby is like suggesting that nobody should eat fats and sugars since excessive fats and sugars lead to obesity and/ or death from heart disease, diabetes or cancer.

In short, McKenna tells us why sleeping with your child is the most biologically normal thing to do and tied to a long and healthy relationship with breastfeeding. His findings are echoed in homes where mothers realize the deep link between the two as they slip into their new role as caregivers. When Bengaluru-based author Dharini Bhaskar became a new mother, she found breastfeeding to be a struggle, but she quickly saw how baby sleep and breastfeeding are entwined.

The first three months were (and remain) a blur. Largely because, for me, it took the whole fourth trimester to finetune the mechanics of feeding my baby at my breast. Once breastfeeding becomes less of a puzzle, baby sleep becomes relatively painless. During the first three months, since I was still to master breastfeeding in the lying down position, and since I hadn't quite grasped babywearing, I'd often hold my son in my arms during naps, and sometimes, through the night. My son was most at ease in my arms, and everything I had read came rushing back. This is how all babies are programmed—they seek proximity with their caregivers. And this is how we, as new mothers, are built—we come with the biological expectation that we will remain bound to our child until he is ready for independence. The key to parent–child happiness in the early months and years is, I believe, that simple: stay close. And this becomes doubly true when each of us is at our most vulnerable—when we sleep.

In hindsight, during the first three months, I'd have worn my baby for his naps—something I came to do recurrently from the fourth month onwards—and learnt, as a matter of priority, the simple art of breastfeeding while lying down. It would have made nights more restful for me.

The Western Bias

In modern times, there has been a pushback against biological norms such as co-sleeping and bedsharing due to what some experts say are 'safety' issues, such as babies being suffocated by blankets or pillows, their parents' bodies, their mother's long, untied hair, and seemingly harmless things in and around the bed. The fact is that both bedsharing and room-sharing must follow all safety rules, such as keeping long hair tied, and not leaving the baby around pillows or loose covers. Parents should also not be inebriated or under heavy, sleep-inducing medication when they sleep with their young ones. When these guidelines are followed, parents are naturally, biologically attuned to keeping their babies safe.

But as McKenna notes, this raising of the alarm against co-sleeping and bedsharing

> stems from an unexpected time in Western history when urban mothers were so destitute that in order for some of her children to live, others needed to be sacrificed in the form of being overlaid . . . Many poor women living in Paris, Brussels, Munich, and London (to name but a few locales)

confessed to Catholic priests of having murdered their infants by overlaying them in order to control family size (Flandrin, 1979; Kellum, 1979; Stone, 1977). Led by priests who threatened excommunication, fines, or imprisonment for actual deaths, infants were banned from parental beds (Stone, 1977). The legacy of this particular historical condition in western history probably converged with other changing social mores and customs (values favoring privacy, self-reliance, and individualism) to provide yet another piece of the overall philosophical foundation at the core of our present contemporary cultural beliefs about sleeping arrangements.

Then come more layers of bias. Fast-forward to the twenty-first century, the Western infants sleep research paradigm 'builds upon negative assumptions about the alleged devastating consequences of co-sleeping behavior,' he adds.

Indeed, so entrenched and often hidden are unproven assumptions and false stereotypes about cosleeping, in whatever form it takes, that contemporary researchers/reviewers reading anti-bedsharing reports are not likely to spot or even notice how and where the authors' cultural assumptions, preferences, and biased interpretations are substituted and passed along as logically deducted scientific truths. These biases prevent researchers from acknowledging that the overwhelming number of deaths in the United States and other western countries involve not cosleeping, but infants sleeping alone.

In effect, these biases, built over a few hundred years, have set a certain 'standard' for sleep trainers to brazenly define how and where infants should sleep. They claim children must be turned into independent sleepers through forced separation in order to offer their parents 'privacy'. The separation, which goes against all biological imperatives, has, therefore, been heavily 'normalized' and termed 'healthy', 'desirable' and 'in the best interests of children and families', so much so that parents following their instincts of attached nighttime parenting are regularly chastised for not doing right by their baby.

Different Cultural Norms across the World

While mainstream Western ideals of how infants should sleep do influence other parts around the world due to greater globalization, the explosion of multimedia platforms and shared parenting literature, they are not the norm in many cultures.

Evolutionary science tells us the human baby, at birth, is the most neurologically immature of primates, with a relatively short gestation period of nine months. The early months after birth are, therefore, called the 'fourth trimester'—when babies benefit from a womb-like atmosphere: close mother–infant contact, skin-to-skin with parents and frequent nursing. This is linked to healthy cardiorespiratory progression and oxygenation, less crying, and better thermoregulation, not to mention the opportunity to establish a healthy breastfeeding relationship.

An interesting paper, 'Exploring Mother-Infant Bedsharing through a Cross-Cultural Lens', in the *Journal of the Motherhood Initiative*, notes:

> Mother–infant sleep arrangements significantly differ in Western and non-Western cultures. In the Western world, mother-infant bed-sharing is often associated with physical

health and safety concerns as well as long-term social/
emotional codependency (Canadian Pediatric Society). In
contrast, mother-infant bed-sharing is often a taken-for-
granted part of the social order in non-Western countries
(Okami, Weisner and Olmstead 244).

Indeed, the cultural practices and social setting of the place
the child is born in or belongs to and the psychology of the
caregivers greatly influence how the child sleeps. In Asian
cultures, it is common for children to sleep with their parents—
unlike in Western countries where separation of the baby
from parents is institutionalized by the medical community.
It's worth considering, as data shows, that higher education
levels, urbanization, economic progress and mothers joining the
workforce have led to a drop in co-sleeping.

A study researching cross-cultural differences in infant and
toddler sleep found that children predominantly from Asian
countries had significantly later bedtimes, shorter duration of
sleep in a 24-hour cycle, and were more likely to room-share
than children from Caucasian regions. These studies also
indicate a difference in certain cultural perceptions such as
forms of protection, the importance of bodily contact between
caregivers and children and family ties.

In Japan, for example, co-sleeping continues to be the
preferred practice, and about 80 per cent of mothers sleep
within an arm's reach of their children. Here, rates of SIDS are
the lowest in the world. In India too, parents tend to sleep in the
same room as their children, where babywearing, breast-sleeping
(as coined by James McKenna, where mothers and infants share
a bed while feeding on demand through the night) and bedsharing is widespread.

In most countries of Europe and large parts of America, by contrast, training babies to sleep in separate rooms is the norm. Of course, even within these regions, there are variations: an interesting study found that Indian-Americans most commonly slept with their babies among ethnic groups in New Jersey and had the lowest rate of sudden unexpected infant death (SUID). 'Conditions that substantially increase the risk of SUID while bed-sharing include smoking, alcohol use, and maternal fatigue,' lead author Barbara Ostfeld, PhD, a professor of Pediatrics at Rutgers Robert Wood Johnson Medical School, was quoted as saying. 'Indian-Americans smoke and use alcohol less than other populations. In addition, grandparents tend to be very active in childcare, which reduces maternal fatigue.'

The practice of bedsharing is as old as our species itself, adds an NPR report, 'Is Sleeping with Your Baby as Dangerous as Doctors Say?' on increasing instances of bedsharing in the US. Homo sapien mothers and their newborns have been sleeping together for more than 200,000 years, the report quotes anthropologist Mel Konner at Emory University as saying. 'Bed-sharing is a tradition in at least 40 per cent of all documented cultures,' Konner says, citing evidence from Yale University's Human Relations area files. Some cultures find it cruel, the report says, to separate a mother and baby at night. 'In one study, Mayan mothers in Guatemala responded with shock—and pity—when they heard that some American babies sleep away from their mothers. "But there's someone else with them there, isn't there?" one mom asked,' says the report in NPR.

The Indian Context

In India, in an average home, shared family spaces that promote kinship and familial bonds trump everything else, and a big family bed that can hold three members, if not four, is at the head of this close relationship. Typically, parents and children room together, the baby nestled in between parents, till she is old enough to move to a mattress on the floor, or demand a separate room. The cot, or a crib, and a nursery (a separate room for the baby) is only a recent entry, as yet a preserve of the Indian elite, a small percentage of Indians who can afford it. On the other hand, it is quite common in Indian homes to put an infant to bed in a traditional sari-cradle, particularly in rural homes. But new evidence warns against this practice to reduce the risk of suffocation as babies are safest when they sleep on flat surfaces.

On the Gentle Baby Sleep India (GBSI) forum, we are often flooded with queries from new mothers about how babies should sleep—which points to a wide gap between modern expectations from baby sleep and biologically appropriate sleep behaviour. We are often asked:

- Is it safer for babies to sleep in a crib?
- My baby doesn't like to sleep in a crib; what should I do?
- Do I really need to separate the baby from me and have him sleep in a different room?
- Should I sleep-train my baby?

The fears of a modern Indian parent are growing every day, under peer pressure to conform to unreasonable expectations that are not in line with the biological imperatives of children. On the other hand, a lackadaisical approach to routines and letting children stay awake beyond exhaustion also leads to increased stress for the whole family. The answer lies somewhere in between, in finding the right balance, which we will get to in the next chapter.

Not all traditional wisdom in India is misinformed, of course. A lot of it is tied to the real needs of children, which many grandparents tend to understand. Elders in India will tell you it's tradition for Indians to hold babies close day and night. This is both a function of economy and attitude: most homes are not large enough to allow for a different room entirely for the baby and do not have the means to have paid childcare. Parents here, as opposed to those in Western cultures, feel a greater sense of safety and control when they have their children within their sight. This does, as we increasingly realize from new evidence and research being conducted across the world, have a deep historical and anthropological basis, something to keep in mind before we fall for claims made by the multimillion-dollar sleep-training industry that feeds on fears and anxieties of new parents and is inching its way to India.

2

The Baby Superpower: Sleep

Sleep is nature's panacea. It restores and nurtures and holds the key to many of your parenting puzzles. Is your child usually cranky? He needs more sleep. Is your child unable to focus on daily tasks? She could do with more sleep. Is your child pushing away his food? Check on his sleep routine. He might be overtired by the time mealtime rolls around. Is your child distracted and uninterested in school or learning? She is possibly underslept. Is your child acting out, throwing tantrums, unwilling to listen to reason, showing signs of behavioural problems? It's most likely linked to sleep and also your choice of parenting. Children who feel that they are respected and their needs taken care of tend to be cooperative.

Sleep is children's superpower. It helps them do better in every aspect of life. After all, the two major engines that drive growth for babies are food and sleep. While most parents are very particular about what they feed their children, sleep is usually grossly neglected, pushed to the back of the routine because so little is known about why it's such an important feature in a child's life.

Sleep is a superpower because it charges babies to be their happiest, most responsive selves. It's what allows them to grow, explore, play, make connections, build relationships, feel creative and express themselves while making them feel like a joyful part of a colourful world. When they are not properly rested, they feel ill at ease, as if something is not right.

Here's a little experiment for you to determine the real power of sleep: Observe a child who sleeps enough for his age and another child who doesn't get enough hours in bed, going by globally recognized guidelines.

A Tale of Two Children

Let's take a peek into 9-month-old Sumer's home. His routine goes like this: he sleeps at midnight and wakes up at 6 a.m., when his mother leaves the bed to get breakfast started. He clocks 6 hours of sleep at night. By the time breakfast is served, Sumer is already cranky and doesn't want to eat. His parents believe that he is generally of a cranky disposition.

By 10 a.m., it's Sumer's bath and massage time. He bawls through both, and his grandmother, who is usually around during the day to assist her daughter in caregiving, concludes that this is how most babies behave when they are bathed. So, nobody suspects something is in fact wrong.

By 11 a.m., Sumer is positively overtired. As he nurses, he falls asleep. Twenty minutes later, his mother puts him down on the bed and, as soon as she moves away, he is up, crying out for her because he finds himself alone and scared. Sumer's mother picks him up and tells her mother that her son hates sleeping. She shrugs—it's probably how all children are. Or maybe it's just her bad luck?

Hours pass and Sumer plays with his grandmother, crying frequently in between as she tries desperately to cheer him up by offering him colourful toys, till around 4 p.m. when he plops off out of exhaustion. His grandmother puts him down on the bed and leaves the room. She tells his mother, 'Look, he sleeps off on his own when he has to! He doesn't need to be helped to sleep.' But Sumer wakes up within 1 hour because he finds himself alone, and crawls out of bed, crying for his mother again.

Throughout the evening, Sumer is awake, taking in the chatter around the house, rubbing his eyes because his nap was too short. He is not able to focus on any fun activity. As the family members gather and get busy with teatime and then dinner prep, he is cranky again, feeling tired and neglected. He cries for attention and seems overstimulated with all the lights on in the house and the television throwing up images that he is attracted to but can't make sense of.

He barely eats at dinner. By the time his mother takes him to bed, it's 10 p.m. But he nurses and fusses at the breast because he is so tired that he is unable to wind down. He slips into a deep sleep only around midnight. By that time, his mother is beyond exhausted. She has no time to herself. She is also annoyed that her husband can't seem to put Sumer to bed.

Sumer's neighbour, Sara, is similar in age. Except that her parents follow an age-appropriate routine which they learnt about through a friend who is a member of GBSI. She goes to bed at 8 p.m. and wakes up at 7 a.m. on her own and that's when her parents leave the bed as she has completed her sleep. She coos happily on her high chair as her father makes breakfast for the family. Her mother takes her to nap the moment she shows the first sleep cues—when her eyes begin to look a bit glazed and droopy and her movements slow down. Her mother notices that she begins to show sleep cues around the same time every day—at about 9 a.m. She sleeps on her lap, and sometimes on the bed, for 45–60 minutes, while her mother catches up on her email and the news.

Sara then plays for the next 3 hours with the house help as her mother gets some work done. When it's time for her next nap, Sara mutters 'Nini', her word for sleep, rubbing her eyes. Her mother takes her to nap immediately. She then naps for the next few hours, with her mother or the helper bridging her sleep in between so that Sara sleeps for 2–2.5 hours and wakes up fresh and ready for the second half of the day.

When Sara goes to the park in the evening with her father, she is full of energy, smiling and trying to blow bubbles at other children. Other parents comment on what a 'happy baby' Sara is, how she readily engages with new people and is usually eager to take in new sights and sounds. Back home, she gobbles down her dinner, listens keenly to her father read a bedtime story and then drifts off to sleep as she nurses with her mother. The day is pretty seamless, save for the odd one and in times of regression or illness.

Notice the difference in how the days unfold at both the homes? The difference is startling. Both sets of parents are responsible and caring and want the best for their children. Both babies were born healthy with the ability to sleep. And yet, because of the difference in the awareness level on the role age-appropriate sleep plays in a baby's routine, both the children are developing very differently.

Sumer is severely sleep-deprived and unable to cope with the stimulations he is offered when he is awake. He resists new experiences and struggles to eat. He either resists sleep, making his parents believe he is a 'poor sleeper', or drops off to sleep on occasion due to exhaustion. Sara is clocking in the recommended number of hours and is developmentally and cognitively doing very well. She is aware of her sleep cues and indicates she wants to sleep at around the same time every day even though she isn't yet a year old. She loves trying new food and is bursting with energy when she is awake.

An Urban Crisis

In Indian cities, sleep deprivation is a serious crisis, and it begins as soon as a baby is born. Most children in India are sleep-deprived, typically going to bed around 10 p.m.–12 a.m., many even later. Parents assume their children do not like to sleep or are poor sleepers. This is highly incongruous because babies are born with the ability to sleep for long hours, as they spend 80–90 per cent of their time in the womb sleeping. Even as they grow into school-going children, they retain the ability to sleep for 10–12 hours a day.

After they are born, infants need 16–18 hours of sleep in a 24-hour cycle. Toddlers need about 13–14 hours of sleep. As children hit the 5–6-year mark, they are able to stay awake longer but still require 10–12 hours of sleep at night to be able to function at their best during the day.

But because so little is known about sleep being as important as food, most parents wonder: what's the fuss about sleep? What's the big deal if a child doesn't sleep the recommended number of hours? Won't the child just fall asleep on his own whenever he feels sleepy?

The shortest answer to the loaded first question is that most brain development in children happens while they are asleep. Millions of neural connections and memories are made and stored and an enormous amount of physical and mental development happens while the body appears to be at rest. Inside a peaceful exterior lying seemingly motionless on a flat surface, the body is nature's most efficient factory at work, doing night duty (and day duty when the child naps!) to make sure you're bright and cheerful the next day. Sleep also has a major role to play in language development, impulse control and strengthening attention spans. When we're asleep, our pituitary gland releases the growth hormone, which aids development and repair.

In a study titled 'Infant Sleep and Its Relation with Cognition and Growth', researchers found 'a positive association between sleep, memory, language, executive function and overall cognitive development in typically developing infants and young children'.

So, you see, there is an overwhelming number of reasons in favour of working on fixing your child's sleep needs (and yours too!). Sleep is your baby's ultimate superpower that will decide how the day will progress. A healthy sleep architecture will help her flourish in every aspect of her day.

What sleep and parenting expert Sarah Ockwell-Smith says in her book, *The Gentle Sleep Book*, resonates with us:

> I firmly believe that the biology of sleep should be taught to all parents. We spend so long learning about labour and childbirth but very little time learning about what happens after the baby is born. If we do, usually all our efforts are focused towards nappy changing, feeding and bathing, but isn't sleep as important? It would be useful if all parents also took a class covering the basics of sleep . . . I have worked with numerous families who see an astounding difference when they have a good grasp on some basic baby biology.

So, in this chapter, we're going to give you a bit of a kickstart to understand all you need to know about the importance and physiology of baby sleep, so you know why it needs to be top priority.

Let's take you through some of the most important aspects of the physiology of sleep.

What Happens When We Sleep?

When we fall asleep, our brain cycles through REM (rapid eye movement) and non-REM sleep. We begin with non-REM sleep or NREM, which is divided into four stages, as we drift off into light sleep. NREM sleep is broken down into three distinct stages: N1, N2 and N3—characterized by larger and slower brain waves. N1 sleep is very light sleep, N2 is increasingly deeper sleep and N3, also referred to as slow-wave sleep, is the deepest NREM sleep stage.

At the light sleep stage, our heart rate and breathing regularizes and body temperature drops. Children at this time are in a very delicate state of sleep—when they easily awaken. We then cycle into a deep sleep, which is considered to be the most restorative part of sleep. As the sleep cycle progresses, we shift to REM sleep, when the eyes move rapidly behind closed lids and we could seem to be back in light sleep, with a faster breathing rate. This is often referred to as the stage in which we dream. But children don't dream until they are about 2 years old (see Box 2.1). Researchers at Johns Hopkins University led by Sleep Expert and Neurologist Mark Wu found that with each cycle, you spend less time in the deeper stages of sleep and more time in REM sleep. Adults cycle through four to five cycles every night, each lasting 70–120 minutes. We spend more time in REM sleep in the second half of the night, which is why you will often find children more likely to wake between sleep cycles then. Children also spend twice as much time as adults in REM sleep.

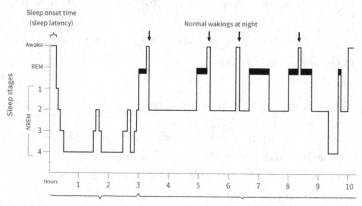

Sleep onset time
(sleep latency)

Normal wakings at night

Deep sleep (NREM 3 and 4)
early in the night

Light sleep (NREM 1 and 2) and dreaming (REM) sleep
during most of the night (REM mainly late in the night)

More deep sleep

NREM Stage 1

(Drowsiness)

- Easily awakened
- Sensation of falling
- Drifting in and out of sleep

NREM Stage 2

(Light sleep)

- Awareness of surroundings fades
- Body temperature drops
- Easily awakened

NREM Stage 3 & 4

(Deep & deepest sleep)

- Most restorative sleep
- Groggy and disorientated if awakened
- Bone, muscle and tissue repair occur
- New growth, appetite regulation and strengthening of memory and immune system take place

REM Stage

(Rapid Eye Movement Sleep)

- The dream stage
- Body becomes immobile
- Transfers short term memory to long term
- Enhances neural connections
- Processes emotions

Infants and children under 3 years of age have shorter sleep cycles, about 30–60 minutes, after which they wake up. As children grow, their sleep cycles become more adult-like, stretching to about 90 minutes by around 5 years of age. Accordingly, it is biologically natural for children to stir briefly after every sleep cycle and need help to enter the next.

This is called 'bridging'. Parents can help bridge these cycles by nursing, rocking, walking or patting. As children mature to about 3–4 years old, they are able to bridge most sleep cycles on their own, falling back asleep without being aware of it, just like their parents.

Wu points to two main drivers of sleep: Circadian Rhythm and Sleep Drive. Let's explore these.

Circadian Rhythm

The Circadian Rhythm is nothing but the approximately 24-hour body clock, determined by the day–night pattern following the movement of the sun. When the sun rises and light filters in, you wake up. When the sun sets and the sky darkens, you begin to feel sleepy. But babies spend weeks, if not months, with little knowledge of night and day. This is because their circadian rhythm has not set in and develops after the first three months. (It's important to note that many babies do have their rhythm in place right from birth.)

Babies whose circadian rhythm hasn't yet set sleep more during the day and may be awake and playful at night. Consistent exposure to natural light and sounds during the day and maintaining a dark and quiet sleep environment at night after month 3 aids this process. Once the circadian rhythm has set in (at around 4 months of age), the sleep environment for day naps has to be kept quiet and dark, as babies become more sensitive to light and sound like adults and might be unable to fall asleep and stay asleep without a conducive environment to suit their changing needs and biological rhythms.

Sleep Drive

Sleep Drive or Homeostatic Rhythm is your ability to fall asleep at a given time based on the sleep pressure created by being awake for a certain period. It is a phenomenon driven by the gradual accumulation of a neurotransmitter called adenosine during the day. Many parents wonder why their babies' day sleep is different from night sleep. Babies typically have lighter sleep during the day and deeper sleep at night. This is because day naps are created by homeostatic rhythms or the body's self-regulating system in which pressure to sleep builds based on how long you've been awake. It's your body's way of ensuring you are getting enough rest, and so, sleep hormones kick in to make you feel sleepy. Night sleep is born of both circadian and homeostatic rhythms; so, the pressure is considerably more enormous, which pushes you towards a big, long, restorative chunk of sleep, lasting about 7–8 hours for adults and 10–12 hours for children.

Powered on Sleep Hormones

In his book *Why We Sleep: The New Science of Sleep and Dreams*, author Matthew Walker says there does not seem to be one major organ within the body or process within the brain that isn't optimally enhanced by sleep (and detrimentally impaired when we don't get enough).

He talks about the powerful role played by the sleep hormone in chief—melatonin.

Melatonin acts like a powerful bullhorn, shouting out a clear message to the brain and body: 'It's dark, it's dark!' At this moment, we have been served a writ of nighttime, and with it, a biological command for the timing of sleep onset. In this way, melatonin helps regulate the timing of when sleep occurs by systemically signaling darkness throughout the organism. But melatonin has little influence on the generation of sleep itself: a mistaken assumption that many people hold. To make clear this distinction, think of sleep as the Olympic 100-meter race. Melatonin is the voice of the timing official that says 'Runners, on your mark,' and then fires the starting pistol that triggers the race. That timing official (melatonin) governs when the race (sleep) begins, but does not participate in the race. In this analogy, the sprinters themselves are other brain regions and processes that actively generate sleep. Melatonin corrals these sleep-generating regions of the brain to the starting line of bedtime. Melatonin simply provides the official instruction to commence the event of sleep, but does not participate in the sleep race itself.

The Main Benefits of Sleep

Sleep is like food, and yet sometimes it's such a silent and underrated feature of our lives that its benefits can seem invisible. Looking at two adults, you can't see the difference between one who grew up eating a healthy diet and one whose diet was less than optimal (unless they are obese or otherwise overtly unhealthy). But internally there can be differences. Nutrition, food, sleep, genetics, stress, environmental factors, physical exercise are all pieces of a jigsaw puzzle that come together to determine a person's overall physical and mental health. Here are some of the areas in which sleep plays a role in children:

- **Growth**

  The growth hormone is primarily secreted during deep sleep and usually in the hours of sleep before midnight—one of the reasons why early bedtime is recommended.

- **Heart health**

  Sleep helps regulate blood glucose as well as the amount of cortisol or stress hormones being produced, hence protecting against vascular damage and diabetes.

- **Obesity**

  Sleep deprivation impacts the production of the hormone leptin which signals to our body that we are full. Without this hormone, we continue to eat. Over time, kids who do not get enough sleep can become obese. Also, tired kids crave high-fat foods (like adults) and they also tend to be more sedentary—all things that lead to unhealthy weight gain.

- **Attention span and cognitive ability**

  Studies have shown that children who consistently sleep fewer than 10 hours a night before the age of 3 are three times more likely to have hyperactivity and impulsivity problems. For school-age kids, research has shown that adding as little as 27 minutes of extra sleep per night makes it easier for them to manage their moods and impulses so they can focus on schoolwork. Children make neural connections and store what they have learned throughout the day in their brains while they are sleeping at night. Naps play an extremely important role in learning too.

The Link between Sleep and Immunity

With the COVID-19 pandemic, the link between sleep and immunity has only been strengthened, with health experts extolling the virtues of clocking in enough sleep to keep your body in top shape.

What exactly is the connection between immunity and sleep? Studies have repeatedly proved that loss of sleep impairs our immune function. This is because when we sleep, our body is busy recovering, repairing and processing the stress and information absorbed through the day. Sleep charges us up to full strength for the next day.

We know that babies need to be fed right for good immunity. But sleep is just as important to build immunity in babies right from birth.

With immature immune systems, young children often fall ill with bouts of fever, cough and cold, especially once they enter school life or come in frequent contact with other children who may be carriers of infection. But age-appropriate sleep can act as a major deterrent to frequent illness. The first few years of life are crucial in developing a strong internal system and robust gut health, and restful sleep is the key. Important hormones are released for growth and development during the time that children are asleep.

The Cytokines Connection

A report by the US-based Sleep Foundation states:

> Without sufficient sleep, your body makes fewer cytokines, a type of protein that targets infection and inflammation,

effectively creating an immune response. Cytokines are both produced and released during sleep, causing a double whammy if you skimp on shut-eye. Chronic sleep loss even makes the flu vaccine less effective by reducing your body's ability to respond.

Lack of sleep also deprives kids (and adults) of natural killer cells and proper immune response, weakening the system. Research has shown that children who do not get adequate naps or who sleep less at night are more susceptible to picking up infections than those who get enough sleep and are well-rested.

As the sun sets, our bodies are biologically designed to wind down, which is why it's important to have an early bedtime for children—to allow the body to follow its natural circadian rhythm. When children are not put to bed at the appropriate hour, their body releases cortisol, the stress hormone, putting the immune function in peril.

Magical Microbiome

For a healthy immune system, you need a fair supply of microbiome, the good bacteria in our bodies, which is directly linked to our circadian rhythms. Put simply, if babies don't sleep enough, their gut bacteria will not be able to digest nutrients from what they eat. In a vicious cycle, poor gut health impacts sleep negatively and leads to sleep loss.

When babies sleep, they heal and grow. Sleep provides the essential backbone to a well-developed immunity for life.

We spend about a third of our lives sleeping. If it wasn't serving a vital purpose, it would be a major goof-up on the part of evolution! In short, help your children power up on sleep and watch them soar.

Box 2.1 Do Babies Dream?

When babies cry in their sleep, or wake up looking terrified, we tend to think they had a bad dream. It turns out that babies do not begin to dream until they are 2 years old. Pioneering psychologist David Foulkes, who studied dreaming in children from the toddler stage to teens in his lab, found that younger children have dreams that resemble static snapshots, like a slideshow, if you will. It isn't until they are 5–9 years old that they begin to dream in terms of moving images. It is closer to ages 7–8 years old that they begin to have proper, story-like dreams, with characters and a narrative arc, as they cycle through REM sleep. Younger children may report dreams, he says, 'often at the prompting of their eager parents'. But the reason that dreams develop at a later stage is that they are tied to the development of the self, consciousness, memory and our place in the world. So, babies, in that sense, are not developmentally ready to begin dreaming.

What do disturb babies are night terrors, often confused with nightmares. You know how sometimes they wake up in terror 1–2 hours after going to bed, unable to calm down even if you soothe them? They are likely to be night terrors that occur when the central nervous system is overstimulated during sleep. This tends to happen when babies are too tired, agitated or late to bed. The best way to deal with it is to keep reassuring the child that all is well and nudge the baby awake if he is unable to calm down. Then gently soothe him back to sleep.

3

How to Get Your Baby to Sleep: The SHARED Method

In the process of helping thousands of parents on GBSI and personally, we have found that there is, indeed, a distinct formula that 'works' to improve infant and toddler sleep. This is not the same kind of 'working' that traditional sleep trainers promise. It will not, in the course of three to four days, lead to a baby sleeping through the night, napping independently and falling asleep on her own in her crib. However, as we will discuss in greater detail later in the book, this picture of ideal baby sleep is in itself flawed and not based on what is biologically normal. It is also the sleep equivalent of a 'fad diet', a quick and dirty effort that leads to short-term, superficial and ultimately harmful results. Our method is the equivalent of a lifestyle change, where one lives by a 'new normal' for around three years. The method is no less miraculous and leads to both immediate improvements as well as long-term health, with good sleep habits and attachment patterns that can last a lifetime. It is based on connection, instinct, biological rhythms and meeting the child's needs. It is a partnership between the parent and the baby and the method is perfectly encapsulated in the acronym SHARED:

Sharing a bed
Holding for naps
Avoiding overtiredness
Routine
Early bedtime
Dark and quiet room

Box 3.1 Gurpriya's Story

For the first year and a half of her son Zorawar's life, sleep was a low priority for Gurpriya Bagga. Zorawar had been in the NICU for two weeks after his premature birth. He weighed 1.7 kg when they brought him home. 'I was trying to get a hold on breastfeeding, bathing and massaging this tiny baby,' Gurpriya reflects. 'Sleep was low on my priority list. On sleep, I had just succumbed. I had no idea about it and it was chaotic. He slept very late at night. I was permanently exhausted. Soon after his first birthday, I was also working and pregnant. It was then, through the Facebook group Breastfeeding Support for Indian Mothers, that I discovered GBSI and everything changed.' Gurpriya then understood that sleep was something that needed to be looked into. She understood concepts like overstimulation and overtiredness. She realized her son's bedtime—midnight—was too late. She began to shift it earlier by 30 minutes every week. Within two months, Zorawar's bedtime had shifted to 8 p.m. and, within three months, to 7 p.m. 'I began to apply the group's tenets,' she recalls. 'I became very protective about his schedule and his bedtime. After that, there would never be an occasion when my mother-in-law, my husband and I would all step out together after 7 p.m.' By the time her second baby, Zoya, was born, Gurpriya knew what to do. She was tandem breastfeeding her toddler and her baby. Although they slept in the nursery with their nanny, Gurpriya found herself spending much of the night in bed with them there because that was what they needed. Zoya was held or worn in a ring sling for all her naps until almost the age of 2 years. 'I received some flak for holding, but I understood the need for it, and so, I did what I needed to do,' she says. 'I kept checking awake windows and age-appropriate routines on GBSI,' Gurpriya says. 'The 2-3-4 schedule worked like a miracle! I was very particular about both food timings and sleep timings as kids thrive on a routine!' Gurpriya found that applying the principles she imbibed from GBSI and making them her own made sleep for both her babies much more manageable and healthy.

Sharing a Bed

Babies sleep well in close physical contact with their parents wherein the parent and the baby can respond to each other's sensory signals and cues. In India, bedsharing is the cultural norm. Bedsharing boosts and eases the breastfeeding relationship. Human milk has a low calorie composition, which is specifically adjusted to the human infant's underdeveloped gut. It requires frequent night feedings, which is facilitated by having your baby within arm's reach. Studies have found that infant responses to maternal smells, movements and touch reduce infant crying and promote better sleep. Proximity to the mother's body helps a baby regulate his breathing, body temperature, absorption of calories, stress hormone levels, immune status and oxygenation.

Human infants are born at a very immature stage of development. They can develop biologically only through continuous contact with, ideally, the mother or, alternatively, another committed caregiver. Staying in light sleep and rousing regularly in conjunction with a caregiver's movements is also safer for newborns as it protects against SIDS. Bedsharing mothers also report more continual sleep as they can attend to their babies without leaving their beds, especially if they are breastfeeding. Professor James McKenna and his colleague Lee Gettler speak of a practice they call 'breastsleeping', where the mother–infant dyad sleeps attached to each other almost the entire night, breastfeeding on and off as the infant needs, with neither of the two ever entirely waking up. In fact, studies have found that the sleep cycles of breast-sleeping mothers and babies synchronize and they enter light or deep sleep stages together and also rouse at the end of sleep cycles together.

Mothers and infants sleeping together is biologically normal—something that can be seen in our evolutionary history, the sleep behaviour of other primates and in cross-cultural sleep arrangements. In Western industrialized societies, a cultural bias against bedsharing has evolved due to a host of historical events (see Chapter 1, 'Sleep in Ancient Cultures'), linking it with infant deaths due to suffocation and promoting a moral value for solitary and independent infant sleep. These biases have then been scientifically validated through studies intended to further promulgate this folk myth. In fact, in many parts of the world, including India, bedsharing is the accepted, expected and instinctive practice. In Japan, Hong Kong and several other Asian countries where bedsharing is the norm, SIDS is either unheard of or its rates are recorded amongst the lowest.

Even in countries where infants are expected to sleep separately—in their rooms or on separate sleep surfaces in the parents' room—researchers have found that what goes on behind closed doors is different from what authorities and health visitors recommend and what parents report officially. Parents do end up bringing their infants into bed with them due to the sheer exhaustion of having to leave their beds repeatedly at night to tend to the babies or due to an instinctive desire to be close to their babies. Regrettably, this also leads to many unsafe practices like falling asleep on a sofa or armchair with their babies.

In her sleep counselling practice, Himani has often found that parents report in their pre-session questionnaires that their babies sleep in cots but, on probing during the session, they admit (with misplaced guilt) to bedsharing for a large chunk of the time. The relief is immense when Himani gives them 'permission' to bedshare and enumerates its many benefits.

Box 3.2 Safe Bedsharing

Bedsharing is perfectly safe if some simple rules (which are really common sense) are followed, including:

1. The mother should ideally be breastfeeding. For the first three or four months, which is the high-risk period for SIDS, bottle-feeding mums should keep the baby on an attached surface and not on the same bed. This is because breastfeeding mums naturally go

into a protective position when sleeping with their infants, called the 'cuddle curl', with their knees bent up, arm tucked under their pillow or head or curled around the baby to make a protective space. There is no way she could roll towards the baby because her legs wouldn't let her. A breastfed baby will instinctively sleep with her face near the breast and will not wander up into the pillows or down under the covers.

2. Both parents should be aware of and in agreement about bed-sharing. Both should consider themselves primary caregivers and be aware of the baby's presence.

3. Infants younger than 1 year of age should not sleep directly next to older siblings.

4. Parents should not be smokers. Both parents (or any parent who is in bed with the baby) should be sober, including free of sedatives and medication, in addition to not being intoxicated by alcohol or drugs.

5. The baby should be a healthy, full-term baby and should always be placed on his back, unswaddled.

6. The bed should be firm and free of extra pillows, heavy blankets, bedding, cords, stuffed animals and gaps.

7. Excessively long hair on either parent should be tied up to prevent infant entanglement.

8. If a parent is obese, he/she can keep the infant in an attached co-sleeper instead of on the bed.

9. The baby should be between the parents or, if the baby is on one side, the bed should be secured with bedrails or pushed against a wall or it should be a floor bed.

Box 3.3 Benefits of Bedsharing

For the Mother	For the Baby
More (in minutes) continual sleep and shorter disturbances	Increased breastfeeding (total minutes and number of nightly feeding sessions)
More restful nights	Clocking more minutes of sleep
Increased sensitization to the baby's physiological status	Less crying time
Sleep stages synchronize with baby's, making nights more manageable and restful	More light-stage sleep, less deep-stage sleep, which is age-appropriate and safer for newborns
More attunement to the baby's cues	More sensitivity to mother's communication
Better milk supply	Better regulation of breathing, body temperature, stress hormone levels, heart rates, absorption of calories, oxygenation, etc.
Longer intervals between births of children (if desired) due to increased prolactin production	Longer breastfeeding relationship

Holding for Naps

Human babies sleep best when in physical contact with their caregivers. They have a biological survival instinct that makes them wake up when they sense separation. This harks back to millions of years ago when the earliest human babies would only survive if they were attached to their parents at every given moment.

Imagine two prehistoric babies. The first baby allows himself to be put down under a bush when asleep. The second baby wakes up and screams and insists on being picked up again. Which baby would be at lower risk of being picked up by a predator or being left to starve? Which type of baby would have a higher rate of survival? Which genetic pool would win the game of evolution? The answer is obvious.

Our babies today have the same biological instincts as those prehistoric babies. They do not know that they are born in a safe condo in Gurugram or a bungalow in Bengaluru. They are biologically programmed to wake if they sense danger, and danger to them is any separation from their caregiver as their survival is entirely dependent on their caregiver.

As we will discuss further in Chapter 5, 'Your Baby's Sleep: 0 to 4 Months', it is quite normal for babies to wake up when they are put down on a bed, and to need holding throughout their nap for most of the first year. In fact, holding for naps follows logically from the discussion earlier regarding the physiological compatibility of mothers and babies sleeping in contact with each other. As research by experts like Professor Helen Ball at the Durham Infancy Sleep Centre has repeatedly shown, mother–infant sleep contact over the first few months of life is simply a logical extension of post-partum skin-to-skin or kangaroo care with consequences for the development of infant sleep biology and maternal feeding physiology much beyond the neonate stage. Touch maintains higher glucose levels in infants, reduces crying, promotes deeper sleep, reduces apneas, and helps to establish a more secure connection with the mother. This is a need that babies outgrow naturally. Nothing that we do can make them achieve this milestone earlier. Some babies may reach it at 4 months of age, needing a caregiver to lie next to them versus holding them in their arms, and some may reach it at 11 months. The best thing to do is to meet our babies' needs and hold them for as long as required. After they are 4 or 5 months old, you can try every two weeks to put them down and see how it goes. If your baby wakes up (either immediately or 10–15 minutes later when the baby cycles into light sleep), you know your baby is not ready. This need usually exists only for daytime naps and not for night sleep (apart from some tricky phases like regressions or teething) as the quality of day sleep and night sleep are very different. Some babies may need holding for daytime naps again during illness or teething or if they are overtired after this milestone is achieved as well.

In fact, 'contact naps' are a very simple and almost magical solution to sleep challenges. A baby who is taking short naps is bound to be in a vicious cycle of overtiredness and it is almost impossible to inculcate long, healthy sleep for such a baby. Meeting this primal, biological need almost instantly transforms your baby's sleep.

Holding a sleeping baby for large chunks of the day is definitely a new normal for all of us. The best way to handle this is to simply embrace it. Be prepared for it and plan for it. When you know it's time for the baby to nap, set up your 'holding station' with everything you need—water, snacks, headphones, books, your phone, a tablet, a TV remote (initially, when the baby isn't disturbed by sound and light). If there is someone to help you at home, they can bring you food or a drink when you need it.

'But how will I ever get anything done?' you might ask. 'I am breastfeeding and, so, it will usually be me holding her and bridging her nap. How will I eat or shower or attend to chores at home?'

You will do all of that when the baby is awake or when someone else is holding her—perhaps for one nap a day. As parents, we often believe that we should 'get things done' when the baby is asleep, but this is not a good idea. It is much more efficient to meet your baby's needs, hold your baby and ensure your baby sleeps well. Then, when the baby is awake, you can hand over a happy, well-rested baby to someone else to play with, or plop the baby into a bouncer, activity gym or, when older, a playpen or high chair near you while you go about your work.

Holding for naps is also a great way for dads to get involved. They can not only do the actual holding, but they can also be the mother's hands and legs—bring her things or do chores for her—if she's the one holding the baby.

The beauty of holding babies for naps is that it forces you—the exhausted parent—to get some rest as well. You can put your feet up, lean back, relax and, if you are on a bed and supported by pillows, even take a snooze. Once your baby accepts being put down next to you for naps, you can take proper naps. This is nature's finely tuned system!

Avoiding Overtiredness

'Keep your baby awake so that she is tired and will sleep better at night!' Sounds logical? Indeed. And yet this common old wives' tale is the opposite of what we should be doing. Counterintuitive though it may seem, it is being well-rested that leads to a greater ability to sleep. In the words of Dr Marc Weissbluth, 'It's not logical, it's biological!'

Of course, there is a logic to it, though it may not seem obvious. When we are tired, our bodies produce a stress hormone called cortisol. This hormone supports the body while it is trying to stay awake and prevents us from sleeping even when it is time to.

To understand this phenomenon, think back to the time when you were in school or college and had to stay up all night to study for an exam. At 3 a.m., you may have begun to feel a little tired. However, by 5 a.m., you most likely felt completely awake, like you had had a cup of coffee (or three!). You may have taken a power nap then or gone straight on to write the exam, returned home and then crashed into bed. When you crashed into bed though, the sleep you entered was most likely not very restful. It would have been a restless, fitful sleep.

So, what exactly happened here? At 3 a.m., when your body became tired but realized that sleep was not forthcoming, it began to release cortisol to keep itself alert and awake. By 5 a.m., the cortisol levels would have been quite high. When you eventually did try to sleep, that cortisol would have kept trying to wake you up, just like a shot of caffeine would.

This phenomenon is the bane of baby sleep. It is extremely important to help our babies fall asleep when we observe early sleep cues. If we miss these cues, our babies' bodies will fill with cortisol and they will suddenly seem awake again—with a second rush of energy that is called the 'second wind' and that misleads us into thinking our babies are not ready to sleep. Soon, our babies and toddlers will become hyperactive and, eventually, cranky. Crankiness is a late sleep cue and a sign of overtiredness. Now, when they try to sleep, the cortisol in their bodies will not only make it difficult for them to fall asleep (leading to immense sleep resistance), it will also keep causing them to wake up or to wake early (and crankily) from their naps. This cortisol will also remain in the body and cause frequent night wakings.

The way to avoid this cortisol production is to observe your child for early sleep cues. It helps to educate ourselves about awake windows—stretches of time that our babies can be awake before they become overtired—at every age so that we know when to watch out for these sleep cues or for times when sleep cues are difficult to read. We will walk you through these cues and awake windows in the chapters that follow. It is also important to help our babies complete their sleep needs, to bridge and extend naps and morning sleep, to ensure that they are fully recharged when they wake, as incomplete sleep also leads to cortisol production.

An overtired baby will neither nap well nor sleep well at night. In fact, an overtired baby is also unlikely to eat well or play well. It can be difficult to see our babies unhappy or under that kind of physical stress. Avoiding overtiredness can lead to a much smoother and happier day for the whole family, which brings us to the next pillar of our sleep strategy: routine.

Routine

Babies and toddlers love predictability. They thrive with some loose structure and rhythm to their days. Considering that they have such little control over their own lives, knowing what comes next gives them a sense of autonomy and comfort.

We do not promote rigid daily schedules with fixed food and sleep timings. What we recommend is a rhythm to the day wherein roughly the same activities follow each other. Sleep schedules based on the baby's cues and awake windows (with adjustments made if a night was choppy or a nap was shorter or longer) rather than fixed timings on a clock help prevent overtiredness as well as resistance to sleep as the baby knows instinctively what to expect. So, for example, a 9-month-old baby's daily routine could look something like this:

- Wake up between 7 and 8 a.m., nurse, go out on the balcony with the caregiver to watch the birds and trees, come back in, spend some time with grandparents and have breakfast.
- Between 9 and 10 a.m., go back into the bedroom and nurse to sleep.
- Wake up around 11.30 a.m. and nurse. Observe chores with mum, like going out to the market in a baby carrier or sitting in a high chair while mum cooks. Have lunch, play in the living room on a playmat.
- Go into the bedroom to nurse and sleep for her second nap between 2 and 3 p.m.
- Wake up from her second nap around 4 p.m. and nurse again. Go with mum to the park or for a baby music class. They return home just as daddy does from work and then it is exclusive time with daddy.
- Dinner is served at 6.30 p.m., after which the baby's bedtime routine starts. Baby nurses to sleep around 8 p.m.

Having this framework in place ensures that the baby gets the sleep and meals she needs, isn't overtired, is well-stimulated and engaged while awake, and the parents also get to plan their chores and work accordingly.

Another element of using predictability to pace our baby's day and help our babies with transitions are 'bedtime routines' and 'pre-nap routines'. It helps to have a series of steps that you take with the baby every day to suggest that night sleep is coming. The length of the bedtime routine depends on the age of the baby. Younger babies usually need shorter routines than toddlers. A good bedtime routine would look something like: a bath or a sponge, a dry or cream massage, changing into pyjamas, saying good night to people and objects around the house, going into a dim bedroom and reading some books and then lights out with nursing or bottle or rocking while playing some music or singing lullabies. Some families may also want to add in prayers.

A bedtime routine signals to the baby's body that night sleep is coming. Dim lighting ensures that the production of melatonin, the sleep hormone, isn't hampered. A routine is also a time of disconnection from the busy world outside and a time of connection with the parent. Studies have found that the parent's emotional availability at bedtime impacts a baby's sleep quality. It is advisable that the routine be conducted by one of the primary caregivers as it is quite a sacred time for the little ones. It helps babies transition into sleep mode and sets the tone for the night.

A similar, shorter sequence before naps is also useful, especially for older babies and toddlers and particularly in phases when they seem to be resisting naps. The baby should be taken into the nap room 15–20 minutes in advance and engaged in an enjoyable, relaxing activity. Reading books is the simplest and most effective. Playing with some quiet toys, doing puzzles or colouring are other options. Then, when the end of the awake window approaches, lights can be turned off, some music turned on and the baby can be rocked or fed to sleep.

Early Bedtime

Early to bed and early to rise leads to a better rested, healthier baby for numerous reasons. In fact, this is how babies' bodies are programmed to sleep if we do not allow modern life to intrude. Children sleep best if their internal body clocks (circadian rhythms) are synchronized with light and darkness outside (the setting and rising of the sun). This means sleeping between 7 and 8 p.m. and waking between 6 and 7 a.m. Children are naturally early risers, so an early bedtime helps them get the required hours of night sleep. Studies have shown that later bedtimes contribute to obesity and other health problems, lower attention spans and alertness, slower cognition, amongst other issues. Growth hormones are also secreted before midnight and so sleep before midnight should be maximized.

A routine based on an early bedtime usually leads to less resistance at bedtime, less disturbed sleep, fewer early morning risings because we avoid overtiredness, and the sleep is more aligned to the baby's circadian rhythms. Contrary to what we may believe, late bedtimes can lead to early morning wake-ups, whereas shifting bedtimes to earlier can often lead to later morning wake-ups and better night sleep overall.

An early bedtime from the very beginning also sets a routine for the child that stands in good stead once school starts. A school-going child who sleeps by 8 p.m. is well-rested and does not need to be 'woken up for school', as has become a sort of cultural norm.

What's more, an early bedtime is easier for the entire family as it gives parents some time for work or leisure and some 'me time' or 'couple time' after the children go to bed. Alternatively, it allows parents to go to bed early and combat some of the sleep deprivation that comes with disturbed nights.

Box 3.4 How to Achieve an Early Bedtime

Dos

✓ Aim for a bedtime between 7 and 8 p.m. by the time the baby is 6 months old.

✓ Start the whole day's routine early so that the age-appropriate number and duration of naps take place.

✓ If bedtime is currently late, shift the whole routine backwards by a few minutes every day to make bedtime earlier.

✓ Expect some variation in the bedtime depending on the age of the baby and the nap schedule. Babies usually have super early bedtimes (even 6 p.m.) immediately after a nap drop and super late bedtimes (even 10 p.m.) just before a nap drop.

✓ Have a predictable, relaxing bedtime routine.

✓ Keep the house dim and quiet for 1 hour before bedtime (preferably 6 p.m. onwards). Make it pitch dark once it is time to sleep.

✓ Give the baby an early dinner to accommodate the early bedtime. It is not unusual for babies to eat dinner at 5.30–6 p.m.

✓ For older babies and toddlers, include enough physical activity throughout the day to reduce bedtime resistance.

✓ Shift quality time with the baby to the early morning instead of in the late evening if you are a parent who returns home late from work.

✓ Ask for support from your entire household to not stimulate the baby 1 hour before bedtime and to support the baby's transition into bedtime. Babies may certainly have FOMO (fear of missing out) about leaving behind excitement in outside rooms, but that needs to be handled with a proper bedtime routine.

✓ Invest in a video baby monitor so that you can step out after the baby is in deep sleep and continue with your evening if you would like to while rushing back in if you see the baby stir so that you can soothe the baby back to sleep. Create a safe sleeping space for the baby with a flat bed, no pillows or loose bedding, a floor bed or bedrails.

Don'ts

✗ Don't necessarily expect an early bedtime before the age of 5–6 months.

✗ Don't wake up the baby in the morning or from naps to shift the routine to an earlier time.

✗ Don't delay bedtime in the hope of a later morning wake-up. That will backfire.

✗ Don't adjust the baby's routine to an adult household routine. Instead, make the household adjust to the baby.

✗ Don't force a baby to stay awake to meet a parent who returns home late from work.

✗ Don't take the baby out for social events or outings if that will delay bedtime.

✗ Don't blindly follow the clock. Follow awake windows. Adjust the baby's bedtime to the end time of the last nap.

✗ Don't wait only for sleep cues as they are easy to miss with younger babies and difficult to identify with older babies. Observe awake windows and stick to your optimal gap between the last nap and bedtime.

✗ Don't keep too many chores for yourself stacked for the evening as that will either delay bedtime or cause stress if you need to stay inside with the baby.

✗ Don't avoid an early bedtime just because you co-sleep and will need to turn in early yourself. Create a safe sleeping space for the baby with a flat bed, no pillows or loose bedding, a floor bed or bedrails. Invest in a video baby monitor so that you can step out once the baby is in deep sleep. In the early months or during growth spurts, you may not be able to step out for very long, but it is certainly possible during much of babyhood and toddlerhood.

Dark and Quiet Room

There is a very simple and yet extremely vital element to managing baby sleep that is often overlooked by parents. After the age of 4 months, babies become increasingly sensitive to light and sound while asleep. It becomes very important to maintain absolute darkness and quiet for your baby's daytime naps and night sleep. Their circadian clocks (day/night patterns) have already formed after the third month and there is no risk of day/night confusion as long as the baby gets plenty of light while awake during the day. Being able to see their environment can be very stimulating and distracting for babies after the fourth month when they become more aware of their surroundings and more social. Something as minor as a dot on a wall or a shadow across a curtain or a caregiver's earring can be endlessly fascinating to babies and prevent them from drifting off into dreamland.

Research has shown that children's eyes are more sensitive to light than adults' eyes, although darkness is recommended during sleep for all humans, including adults. It's important to remember that light, especially at night, is a modern phenomenon that has come up after the invention of electricity in the twentieth century.

During the night, darkness stimulates the pineal gland to release melatonin, the sleep hormone. Even a small amount of light can obstruct this release.

If the room is pitch dark, babies fall asleep faster and more easily and also re-settle between sleep cycles more easily—both during naps as well as at night. Many parents report a magical transformation in their baby's sleep after implementing this one change. In fact, in Himani's professional practice, 100 per cent of parents who have implemented pitch darkness diligently have experienced an immediate and dramatic change in their babies' sleep.

Box 3.5 Frequently Asked Questions about Implementing the Magic Darkness Sleep Cloak

How do I make it pitch dark?

Curtains and blinds are usually not sufficient as light leaks from under them and around them. The simplest way is to stick layers of black chart paper, newspaper or aluminium foil on the windows. If the room can be designated a sleeping room and the baby can spend time in other rooms while awake, this window covering can be permanent. Otherwise, Velcro can be used to create a removable covering. Block light from electronics (ACs, purifiers, plug points) with black tape. At night, switch off any night lights, zero-watt bulbs or lights in adjoining rooms that may leak in from under doors.

How do I prepare bottles/change diapers, if needed?

Please use a red light focused only on the area needed and not one illuminating the whole room. Red light is the least obstructive to melatonin release but it does not solve the stimulation problem so please do not leave it on any longer than necessary. A mobile phone torch can also be used if it's a matter of a minute or two.

Will my baby be afraid of the dark?

Babies find darkness extremely comforting. They are used to darkness in the womb. They are not afraid of the dark until they reach preschool age, if at all then. A fear *could* develop if toddlers are told scary things about the dark or if they wake often and are not attended to immediately. Bedsharing children are less likely to be afraid even then as they have physical proximity to a parent.

A baby who cries when the lights are switched off when it's time to sleep is most likely resisting sleep and not afraid of the dark. The light being switched off is a clear indication that now it is sleep time. A baby who seems anxious when she wakes in the middle of the night is also more likely to be resisting going back to sleep or resisting the mode of being put back to sleep (for example, if we are rocking the baby, but the baby wants to be fed to sleep). Of course, when the light is switched on, the baby calms down as she gets distracted and sleeping ends for the time being. Parents could misunderstand this to be a preference for light over darkness.

So, it is important to note that we often mistake other issues for a dislike of the dark. However, if, after considering all these options, you still feel your toddler or preschooler (not baby) doesn't like the dark, you can address this in various ways. Play games with a torch—such as shadow puppets or 'dark room'. See if you are comforting the baby quickly enough and if the baby is feeling your touch immediately upon waking. At the end of the day, the benefits of using darkness will most likely outweigh any benefit of having light.

Will I be able to check on my child?

Yes, you will, as your eyes will adjust. You will also be physically aware of your baby next to you. Your baby needs to be in a safe sleep setting in any case as you are not checking on your baby when you are in deep sleep. If needed, switch on the screen of your cellphone or a mild torch/red light for a few seconds for a quick check.

The SHARED method is a highly effective strategy to help your baby sleep well. It has already helped thousands of parents instil longer, healthier, age-appropriate naps for their babies and foster longer stretches of night sleep in which a baby hardly ever wakes fully. It does not involve any distress to babies or parents and is completely aligned to biological rhythms and instincts.

Sleep management based on SHARED principles can lead to a dramatic change in your baby's sleep and much more joy, rest and connection as a family.

Box 3.6 Gurpreet's Story

Gurpreet Kaur became a member of GBSI when her son, Viraj, was around 3 months old. Gurpreet was very troubled by the fact that her baby was unable to sleep in his cot for his daytime naps. 'He would sleep in his cot just fine at night but not during the day,' Gurpreet recollects.

'I had noticed even before joining the group that he would sleep a lot better if I held him or kept him on me but everyone around me started admonishing me, saying that I was spoiling him, that I should swaddle him, place him in a jhula, and so on. Somehow, all of this advice did not sit well with me. I had also googled a lot and read about how my baby should always be kept separate from me, that bedsharing can be a SIDS risk, that I should put my baby down drowsy but awake so that he learns to sleep independently, that I should let him cry. Not only did advice like 'drowsy but awake' not work when I tried it, but it also sounded wrong to me. Then, I joined GBSI and, for the first few days, I just scrolled through the posts. There was a lot of information and it took me a while to sort through it all. By then, Viraj was three-and-a-half months old and had hit the sleep regression phase. But, having read a lot on the group page, I learned what to expect and I was prepared. The first thing I did was that I stopped putting him down in his cot. I kept him next to me in bed or I held him in my arms. Bed-sharing, breastfeeding, nursing lying down were all game-changers for me. We sailed through the 4-month sleep regression.'

Gurpreet found that following the basic principles of the group—bedsharing, holding, following awake windows, maintaining a dark room—actually made her baby's sleep a non-issue for her. She could count the bad nights on her fingers. 'There was a huge conflict between the advice I was generally receiving or reading about on the Internet and what my baby seemed to be telling me,' Gurpreet says. 'GBSI made me understand what was normal and their reassurance permitted me to meet my baby's needs. It also helped me put practices in place that supported my baby to sleep better the way his body is designed to.'

Gurpreet reports that her main focus became maintaining Viraj's awake windows and she would not compromise on them at any cost. Initially, she observed for early sleep cues, but as he grew and became more active, she found it easier to follow awake windows than to spot the cues. 'Once I started noticing how much they matter, I became particular about them. They are like a magic wand!' she exclaims. The awake windows not only helped Viraj sleep better but also helped Gurpreet plan her day and brought predictability and routine to her life.

Gurpreet held Viraj for naps until after the 4-month sleep regression kicked in. Then, she would gently place him next to her on the bed. By the time he was 8 months old, she could even step out for short stretches since she knew how long his sleep cycles were and when she would need to bridge his naps.

Gurpreet works full time (from home during the pandemic) as a content manager for an educational institute. She found that she could work much more efficiently if she followed all the recommendations on GBSI and if Viraj was sleeping well. Since she needed to support him and parent him when he was sleeping, she mostly worked when he was awake. Of course, she could send emails while he slept or attend virtual meetings in which she did not need to speak. However, she would schedule all meetings that required her active participation during his awake periods. Viraj's father or Gurpreet's in-laws would care for him while he was awake. She would schedule work over the weekend as well when her husband was available to take care of Viraj so that she could catch up on work.

Gurpreet admits that regressions are difficult.

'We all need to accept this and understand that it is going to take time, maybe two to three weeks, though it has been even longer for me,' she says. 'But, if you follow the tips and tricks given on GBSI, things become easier. You know that once the regression passes, your baby is going to sleep just fine. If you start giving up and thinking you just can't manage your baby's sleep, then nothing is going to help you and then your baby will enter a cycle of overtiredness. You need to hold your baby for naps, ensure the room is pitch dark and follow awake windows. It is as simple as that.'

Gurpreet has not maintained an inordinately early bedtime for her baby, like 6.30 p.m. or 7.30 p.m., but Viraj has always slept between 8.30 and 9.30 p.m. and earlier during nap transitions. This worked for her because her room has always been quite dark and hence Viraj has not been a particularly early riser. 'My room had only a tiny window, which was covered, so there was hardly any light in the room in the early mornings or for daytime naps,' Gurpreet shares.

'During the 8-month sleep regression, we blocked any little specks of light as well. Pitch darkness works like magic. I have struggled on the few occasions when we have been outside of our home and I have needed to make him nap. If there is visibility in the room, I have to hold more and bridge more. I have no problem with meeting his need for darkness because I understand that he is currently in a phase wherein he is distracted by everything around him. When he is 3 or

4 years old, he might not remain so sensitive to light. I sleep better in pitch darkness, so why wouldn't he?'

After understanding the SHARED Method from GBSI and applying the tenets methodically in her own life, Gurpreet understood the value and efficacy of these simple practices. She soon began to advise other parents on their queries and became a peer counsellor on the group.

4

What Baby Sleep Looks Like: The Sleep Pyramid

Pranay and Gauri had fallen into a beautiful routine with their 7-month-old son, Kartik. The baby would wake around 6.30 a.m. and his father would take him out to the terrace for some morning sun while his mother slept in for a while. After some time in a baby carrier looking at the trees, Kartik would play on a mat while Pranay had his morning coffee. Pranay would sometimes carry Kartik to the bedroom after this for a quick 'swig' of breastmilk from his sleeping mother. After that, Kartik would spend some more time with his father and the nanny, playing with stacking toys or flipping through (and mouthing!) books. At around 8 a.m., Pranay would take the baby back to the bedroom, lay him next to Gauri and the baby would peacefully nurse to sleep for his first nap, waking from that about an hour later. Pranay would then get ready and leave for work.

Feeling quite refreshed from this morning stretch of sleep after a night peppered with brief wakings, Gauri would now rise with her son and they would both have breakfast. Then she would bathe the baby and, by 11.30 a.m., it would be time for

Kartik's second nap. Gauri would nurse him and then usually hold him for this nap while she either dozed or listened to an audiobook. He would wake by 1.30 p.m. After a shower and lunch, Gauri would spend some time playing with him. At 4 p.m., Gauri would nurse him to sleep and then transfer him carefully to the nanny's arms and step out of the room. She would attend to her work until the baby woke again by 5 p.m. She would then take him out to the park for a while or to visit his grandparents. By 7 p.m., it would be time for his bedtime routine and, by 8 p.m., he would be asleep for the night.

However, when Kartik turned 8 months old, this graceful rhythm suddenly got dislocated and it only seemed to get worse. He was not falling asleep easily for his naps and was waking early from them. He seemed to resist sleep at any given time of the day. His bedtime got delayed to as late as 10 p.m. He sometimes took short naps and went to bed early, waking for 1–2 hours at night or very early in the morning. He was cranky and clingy all day. He sometimes needed to be held for long stretches at night as well.

It took about a month for them to settle into a routine again. Eventually, Kartik began to take two long naps, instead of three shorter ones. Gauri and Pranay had read about the golden '2-3-4' pattern on GBSI and their baby had fallen into it naturally. He had gone through a burst of developmental leaps as well. After a rocky few weeks, the family was in a harmonious rhythm again.

Parents of young babies will recognize this pattern of harmony and disharmony, of calm followed by a storm followed by calm again, and of sleep becoming 'chunkier' as babies grow. In this chapter, we are going to talk about the three phenomena that cause this to happen.

Consolidation of Sleep

Babies change every few weeks in every area of development. We as parents are usually familiar with the main physical and cognitive milestones. They smile when they are 2 months old. They sit up at 6 or 7 months old. They start crawling at 9 months old. They wave bye-bye around the same time. They start walking anywhere between 9 and 17 months. As the baby's brain grows, she seems like a completely new person every few weeks. That adorable quizzical newborn look gives way to laughing out loud at 4 months. At 7 months, babies can transfer objects between hands. At 10 months, babies understand that an object they cannot see still exists somewhere. By 12 months, their brains have doubled in size since birth. By 18 months, babies communicate by using single words. They hand toys to us to play with. They begin to follow stories in books. They enjoy imitating adult life with toys. By 2 years old, they can build towers, throw balls, understand two-step instructions and follow complex stories. The age of 3 years is a major milestone when they become capable of reasoning to quite an extent. They separate more easily from parents or caregivers, take turns in games, carry on conversations, undertake problem-solving with buttons and levers, construct simple puzzles and create elaborate make-believe games.

Isn't it miraculous how they leap and grow? In much the same way, baby sleep patterns too unfold like a blossoming flower—but parents are less familiar with this evolution. The first three years of life see distinct phases of sleep. Sleep patterns consolidate and evolve as the months pass. These phases are linked to neurological development, and sleep milestones are as important as developmental milestones like crawling, walking and talking. If we expect our 4-month-old to take only two long naps in the day, versus four small ones, we are expecting something that occurs at the same stage as crawling! If we expect our 6-month-old to sleep through the night, we have jumped ahead by almost 3 years.

As newborns, babies take several short and long naps. This broken sleep starts to consolidate as the weeks pass. By 3 months, there is a long chunk of night sleep plus several small naps. By 4 months, there is a fairly predictable pattern of five naps in addition to a long night sleep. Naps keep merging as the baby becomes older. We call this the Baby Sleep Pyramid.

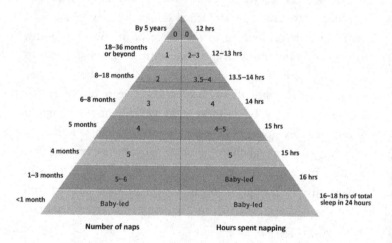

Although the hours of total sleep do not change very dramatically, the 'blocks of sleep' reduce. By 18 months, babies are taking only one nap of 3 hours in the day and sleeping 11 hours at night. By 3–4 years, many babies have stopped napping during the day and get their 12 to 12.5 hours of sleep at night itself.

'But, wait, every baby is different, right?' we hear you ask. Well, yes, babies are different, but they are also not *that* different. Their neurological development does follow the same broad timeline. Some milestones have tighter timelines and some are broader. A child may start sitting without support anywhere between 5.5 and 7 months, but can start walking anywhere between 9 and 17 months! Similarly, a baby will shift to taking three naps in the day anywhere between 5 and 6.5 months, but will transition to taking only a single nap in the day anywhere between 14 and 22 months. However, the transition to three naps will not happen at 8 months! And the transition to a single nap will not happen at 11 months.

Just the way we would not expect our 5-month-old to start running and talking, it's important for us to understand how a 5-month-old sleeps, and not have unreasonable expectations. Once we know what to expect, we will be able to observe our baby's sleep cues and create a predictable routine.

Two types of 'events' in our babies' development push this process along, usually in a two-steps-forward, one-step-back sort of way. These are sleep regressions and nap transitions.

The Regression Conundrum

Maya's daughter, Ira, was 3 months old. After waking every hour or two through the day and night for her entire newborn life, she had suddenly started sleeping long stretches. Maya would wake up in the morning in a pool of milk as her daughter hadn't woken to feed for the last 6 hours. She would check on her with some mild panic and find her sleeping peacefully. As the days passed, Maya started to count her lucky stars and feel an understandable maternal pride. She had lucked out and been blessed with a miracle baby who slept beautifully! She bragged about it on her mommy WhatsApp group and her Instagram page. She felt like a new person after getting these long stretches of sleep.

Then, suddenly, when Ira was 3 months and 3 weeks old, almost overnight, something changed. Ira started waking up every hour at night. Her naps became short. She became cranky and fussy and impossible to soothe to sleep. While Ira would be awake and playing in an activity gym in the middle of the night, Maya started googling frantically through bleary eyes: '4-month-old not sleeping'.

As she discovered soon enough, Ira had hit that most notorious of sleep milestones, the 4-month sleep regression, and this was only the first of many more. Ira's sleep would never be the same again.

The first two years of a baby's life are punctuated by sleep regressions—periods of disturbed sleep and increased night wakings caused by intense skill-building. Regressions occur at times of immense mental and physical development and, as such, the term 'regression' can be misleading as it seems to connote the opposite. The thing is that when babies are undergoing such huge transformation, their sleep deteriorates and seems to regress. Hence, sleep *regresses* while the baby *progresses*.

Some sceptics point out that there is no scientific evidence behind sleep regressions. While it may be true that specific studies identifying every single sleep regression have not been conducted, there *are* studies that link developmental leaps with sleep disturbances. Arguing over the term 'sleep regression' is just semantics. The condition may not be medically diagnosable, but the idea that developmental leaps and emotionally difficult periods cause sleep disturbances is logical, has been studied and is also verified through thousands of anecdotal accounts worldwide and on GBSI itself.

Physical milestones like learning to crawl or walk or talk, cognitive growth like starting to form word associations and then talk, and emotional milestones like developing separation anxiety all contribute to these sleep disturbances. This is often accompanied by teething or growth spurts, which add to the trouble. Very often, though not always, babies drop a nap at the end of a sleep regression, which requires its own form of management.

Here are some of the common signs of sleep regression:

- More wakings to feed or be soothed at night
- More active night wakings
- Increased fussiness during naps
- Increased fussiness during feeding sessions
- Short naps resulting in more crankiness
- Need for holding in arms throughout naps or at night
- More frequent bridging of naps
- Early morning wakings.

The peak period of a regression cycle usually lasts two to three weeks. This can be a very trying time for parents, but it behoves us to remember that it is, in fact, equally tough, if not tougher, on the baby. The best way to cope with it is to go with the flow—without imposing a routine on them. This does not mean, of course, that we don't offer any structure or support and allow them to get overtired as that will only make matters worse. We should observe their cues and meet their needs. If the baby wakes early in the morning, start the nap earlier, hold through the nap and try to extend it. If naps are short, offer an additional nap or shift bedtime earlier. Catch early sleep cues to avoid overtiredness but also keep an eye on their awake windows as cues can be difficult to observe if they are highly stimulated and distracted. The rule of thumb would be: follow early sleep cues or the end of the awake window, whichever comes first.

It helps to have a menu of ways to support their sleep. A baby who was earlier just nursing to sleep or being rocked to sleep may not fall asleep that way any more. Nursing, rocking, bottle-feeding, walking in a baby carrier, taking them for a drive all need to be tried, and the first three in pitch darkness. Playing music while carrying out the soothing can be immensely powerful. It should be music that your baby enjoys and not necessarily conventional lullaby music. Babies often prefer full musical sound with a good beat. A new song that captivates the baby's interest and allows you to soothe her can be a lifesaver during a sleep regression.

Do everything in your power to preserve their sleep. If you were no longer holding your baby throughout naps, you may need to go back to doing that during sleep regressions to ensure that your baby sleeps long stretches. Go the extra mile to ensure that you bridge their sleep cycles. Stay with them while they nap or watch them on a video monitor so that you can soothe them back to sleep in a heartbeat when they stir. If you aren't doing so already, start making it pitch dark and quiet for both daytime naps and night sleep. Blacken your windows completely during the day and stop using night lights.

Finally, be aware of the possibility of dropping a nap. If the sleep regression coincides with a nap transition, it usually settles once the nap routine stabilizes once again. This brings us to the third sleep leap.

Box 4.1 What Are Active Night Wakings?

What we call active night wakings are basically occasions when a baby wakes up at night and is not easily soothed back to sleep, so, she wants to wake fully and play. These are different from the normal wakings that are a few seconds or minutes long—like at the end of a sleep cycle—where a baby is easily soothed back to sleep through feeding or rocking or, when they are older, with a cuddle. If active wakings occur towards the early morning hours, say at 5 a.m., they can sometimes be misunderstood by parents to be an early rising whereas babies actually need to be soothed back to sleep and the waking needs to be handled in the same way as an active waking.

Active night wakings are different and can be much more exhausting for both babies and parents. After the age of 4 months, when a baby's circadian rhythms have formed and the baby has some concept of day and night, a baby will not usually wake to play at night. If she does, it means something is going on. One possibility is that the baby does not have an age-appropriate sleep schedule—meaning, the right number and length of naps, optimum gaps between naps or a suitably early bedtime. Another is that the sleep environment is not conducive—it isn't pitch dark and quiet or the temperature is not comfortable. It is also possible that the baby is going through a nap transition or a sleep regression.

How should you handle active night wakings? When the baby wakes up at night (or very early in the morning), continue to keep the room dark. You can soothe the baby with your voice and shush her as you try to make her sleep again by feeding or rocking. If the baby does not fall back asleep in about 30 minutes, you may need to throw in the towel and let her play for a certain amount of time before once again soothing her back to sleep. It's important to analyse the reason for the active night waking to figure out how to deal with it.

Nap Transitions: How Things Get Easier

From taking multiple small naps as newborns, babies start to consolidate their sleep and, by the time they are 1 year old, are usually taking two predictable naps in a day. Moving from four naps to three to two to one and then finally giving up napping altogether by the age of 3–5 years is a biological process that needs frequent parental intervention and sleep management. From the chaos of the early days, with each nap transition, all the pieces of the baby sleep puzzle begin to fall into place and the baby's and the parents' day starts to take on a lovely, natural rhythm.

Srinivas got in touch with us when his twin girls, Saisha and Maira, were 1 year old. Until then, they had been following the golden '2–3–4 pattern'. Suddenly, they were resisting their naps with all their might. Saisha had stopped taking her second nap altogether. Srinivas insisted that he knew his daughters, that not all babies were the same and that it was time to shift them to one nap. We explained that there is a sleep regression at 12 months linked to the walking milestone and that babies very often resist naps in this phase. We suggested a few ways, as mentioned above, that would help them ride out the regression. We also advised him to expand the awake windows a bit. Srinivas was not in touch for a while after that. When his daughters turned 15 months old, he got back to us with the report that they had, in fact, reverted to two naps with longer awake windows for many weeks. However, the trouble had recently returned. Since most babies do drop from two naps to one between 15 and 21 months, we then guided him on how to navigate this transition, including the 16- and 18-month sleep regressions. He and his wife, Kamala, worked on helping their babies sleep longer for their first nap, which would allow them to drop the second nap and move to an early bedtime of 6 p.m. This is a lengthy transition and it was only by 19 months that Saisha and Maira had truly shaken off the second nap. Srinivas, Kamala and the girls had now regained a routine and the parents raved about how predictable their days had become. The twins woke up at 7 a.m., napped from 11 a.m. to 2 p.m. and went to bed between 7.30 p.m. and 8 p.m. The family was able to plan its day, including afternoon outings, a few music and sensory classes for the toddlers in the early evenings and a reasonable bedtime that gave the parents time to themselves at night.

Nap transitions can be tough experiences, but they lead to a much more settled and predictable routine. The first few transitions occur in quick succession as babies shift from five to four to three naps within the first 6 months itself. Thereafter, transitions move farther apart from each other and also take longer to resolve. The transition from three to two naps takes place between 8 and 10 months; the transition from two naps to one nap takes place between 15 and 21 months, as in Srinivas's case above, and can take 2–3 months to settle down. The final transition, from taking one long afternoon nap to no nap at all, takes place anywhere within the vast span of 3–5 years and can take 6–8 months to be complete.

How do we know if it is time to drop a nap? Like with all things linked to sleep, your baby will tell you, if you know how to listen! Your baby will start to resist naps and bedtime despite everything being in place from your end. Naps will become short. There will be early morning wakings and active night wakings.

These will ease as you start to expand their awake windows, meaning, take them for their naps and bedtime a little bit later every few days. Eventually, the last nap of the day and bedtime will be occurring so late in the day that it will make sense to

Sleep Requirements by Age

Months	Total sleep (hours) Higher figure for younger babies and decreasing until next nap drop	Number of naps	Hours spent napping Higher figure for younger babies and decreasing until next nap drop	Awake windows Increase as day progresses—consider lowest figure before first nap and highest before bedtime	Night sleep length Higher figure for younger babies and decreasing until next nap drop
<1	16–18	Baby led	Baby led	5–30 minutes	No concept of day and night
1–3	16	5–6	Baby led	From 30 minutes at 1 month to 75 minutes at 3 months	Circadian rhythms form by month 3. 10–11 hours after that
4	15	5	5	45–90 minutes	10–11 hours
5	15	4	4–5	1 - 2.5 hours	10–11 hours
6–8	15	3	4	1.5–3.5 hours	10–12 hours
8–18	13.5–14	2	3.5–4	2–4 hours (2–3–4 pattern)	10–12 hours
18–24	13–14	1	3	4–5.5 hours	11–12 hours
24–36 or beyond	12–14	1	2–3	4–7 hours	10–12 hours
After dropping all naps (3 to 5 years)	12	0	0	12 hours	12 hours

drop that last nap and shift bedtime to a (somewhat unearthly) early hour like 6 p.m. It is not unusual for babies to sleep 12–13 hours at night immediately after dropping a nap and then wake up at 6.30 a.m. or 7 a.m. the next morning.

We will now talk about every step of the sleep pyramid in greater detail in the next chapters: what sleep looks like at this age, what changes take place in sleep physiology, age-appropriate soothing methods, the sleep regressions and nap transitions that occur and some of the unique challenges we might face at every stage.

5

Your Baby's Sleep: 0 to 4 Months

The Fourth Trimester

Human babies are born at a very dependent stage. They are, in fact, practically extensions of their mothers (or other primary caregivers) for quite a long time. You may have heard the phrase 'the fourth trimester', coined by anthropologist and midwife Sheila Kitzinger in 1975 and popularized by several parenting experts thereafter, referring to the first 3 months after birth as an extension of the three trimesters of pregnancy, when it helps to think of babies as still at a gestational and heavily reliant stage. At this stage, babies sleep almost the entire day, and their greatest need is for *physical connection* with their parent.

Why are human babies born at such an immature stage? As we know, human beings evolved from walking on all fours to walking on two legs millions of years ago. The human head, containing the large human brain, is quite large relative to the rest of the human body and needs to be able to go through the narrow pelvis of a biped. For this to happen, a human baby needs to be born at an early stage, when it is still small.

The womb is a perfect, constant environment. Babies are tightly cocooned in a warm, dark, cosy place. They don't experience hunger or thirst. They don't need to feed or pass wind or burp. Poo and pee get automatically cleaned up. They are lulled to sleep with gentle rocking and muffled sounds. They know that they can sleep without a care in the world, completely and utterly safe, fulfilled and at no conceivable risk.

When they leave the womb, suddenly everything is very, very different. They feel air and space around them. There are bright lights and loud sounds. They can be moved from place to place. They need to ask to feed. They are suddenly at the mercy of all kinds of unnamed and unseen dangers. In this scenario, they feel safe only in the arms of a caregiver or feeding from the mother's breast.

Babies today are the same as they were millions of years ago. A baby who allowed himself to be left under a bush would be at much higher risk of death from predators or starvation than a baby who screamed to be picked up by the caregiver as soon as he was put down. The ones who clung to their parents had a much higher rate of survival and so those are the babies that exist today. They are biologically programmed to cleave to their caregivers—like the little monkey babies we see holding onto their mammas as they swing from tree to tree. And, so, that is how human newborns sleep best: wrapped to their caregivers, physically connected, with regular rocking and feeding.

This dependence does not end at 3 months. Research theorizes that the 'gestational' phase outside the womb lasts well into the second year. For human babies to reach the same developmental stage that many other mammals are born at, human pregnancies would need to be 18–21 months long, instead of the current 9!

Moreover, species with large brains and high intelligence across the animal kingdom have a long dependent period—a 'childhood'. Take birds, for example. Some species of birds, like chicken, geese and turkeys, are quick to mature but are not very intelligent. Other species, like crows and parrots, have a long period of dependence on their parents when they grow their brains and learn skills. They are exceptionally intelligent. Is it surprising then that human beings, who are at the far end of the intelligence, learning and brain size spectrum, are also at the extreme end of the dependence and immaturity scale? Human children need care, attention and parental investment for a long time and it starts with the intense holding, feeding and soothing required by babies.

What Does Sleep Look Like Now?

Babies sleep and feed all day and the two are intricately linked. They feed to sleep and they wake to feed. Awake windows (the amount of time a baby can remain awake before becoming overtired) are extremely short. They need to be held a lot. They usually wake up if put down on a bed. They nurse very frequently. They need a lot of rocking. They wake frequently at night and feed for both hunger and comfort.

In the first two months, babies have no concept of day and night. Though babies do receive some of the sleep hormone, melatonin, in the womb and from breastmilk, their circadian rhythms develop in the third month. Bedtimes are often quite late—even 2 or 3 a.m.—and shift earlier as the months progress.

Before they are 1 month old, babies sleep about 16–18 hours in the day and their awake windows are extremely short, at between 5 and 30 minutes. The windows increase to about 75 minutes in month 3 and about 90 minutes in month 4. They are shortest at the beginning of the day and longest just before bedtime, though a shorter than usual nap may lead to a short awake window immediately after.

Evening Fussiness, Cluster Feeding and Growth Spurts

Evenings can be difficult with newborns, earning them the daunting moniker 'the witching hour'. Babies may nurse for a few minutes, pull off, fuss and cry, nurse again. Or they may refuse to nurse and refuse to sleep. It may seem as though nothing will soothe them. They also cluster feed—meaning, nurse almost continuously for several hours. They usually have their longest stretch of sleep after this. Sometimes, this evening fussiness crosses over into what some doctors call 'colic'—the infamous, unexplained phenomenon of a baby crying for three hours per day, three times a week for more than three weeks.

There are several theories on what causes this evening fussiness. The first scapegoat, of course, is breastfeeding—we often hear people around us saying, 'the baby is not getting enough milk', and then suggestions for offering top feeds begin. However, this is usually not the case. Babies do cluster feed and nurse very frequently. They could be tanking up their little bellies for the night ahead. They could be overstimulated and overtired from the day's happenings. They might be remembering mum being active at this time during her pregnancy and want to be held, rocked and nurtured in the same way. Interestingly, anthropologist Dr Katherine Dettwyler, who researches breastfeeding in traditional societies, has found that babies in Mali, West Africa, and other traditional societies don't have colic or evening fussiness. These babies are usually wrapped up to their parents all day, nurse several times an hour and sleep on demand.

Here are some ideas on how to soothe your baby during the witching hour:

- Offer to nurse often
- Burp the baby and check for gas
- Soothe with sound—play music or white noise, shush or hum while walking or rocking
- Soothe with rhythmic motion—rock or sway with music or humming
- Wear the baby in a sling or carrier
- Change the caregiver as babies sometimes respond differently to a new touch and the primary caregiver sometimes just needs a break. This is a great time for daddies to step in and walk, rock or play with the babies.
- Go outside. Many babies calm down instantly outdoors.
- Reduce stimulation by lowering light levels, the number of people and noise.
- Try a gentle massage or a warm bath if the baby likes them.
- Vary the nursing position or try nursing in motion.

It's important to keep in mind that during the tough phases of baby sleep—from the witching hour during the newborn phase to sleep regressions later—we should have a menu of ways in which to soothe the baby. You can even pin a checklist to a door or on the fridge to run your eyes over when you're caught in a particularly difficult moment when the baby won't stop crying and you can't think straight. Often, something that worked before stops working and we need to try a new method or even a combination of methods. The newborn phase is when we as parents go through the learning curve on this.

In this stage, babies also go through frequent growth spurts. They feed more frequently and sometimes also sleep more to help their bodies and brains grow. They may be clingier or fussier during these phases. They may pull all-nighters on the breast. It's important to feed on demand in this phase and help babies sleep as much as they need to. It is common for parents to introduce a bottle during a growth spurt as the baby's appetite may seem insatiable, but this is a bad idea. By nursing more, babies are increasing the mother's supply to their needs. The best approach is to feed on demand, eat well and hydrate well. The growth spurt will pass.

Early Sleep Cues

The newborn phase is all about learning your baby's language. What is the baby trying to communicate? Identifying different types of cries is one way. And then there are cues. Just the way 'feeding on demand' involves observing for early hunger cues, proper sleep management means discerning early sleep cues. It is very important to help our babies sleep when we see these early signs of tiredness. These can include blank stares, rubbing eyes and ears, averting their gaze, turning their heads (see chart).

Infant Sleep Cues

Phase One 'I am a little sleepy'	• Averts eyes • Turns head • Blank stare • Rubs eyes
Phase Two 'Ready for bed now'	• Yawns • Sneezes • Frowns • Roots for feed

Phase Three	• Arches back
'Overtired'	• Cries
	• Falls asleep abruptly
	• Fusses during feed

Let's say that you observe the early sleep cues of your 2-month-old about 30 minutes after she woke from her last nap and decide to quickly use the bathroom while your mother distracts the baby. When you return, your mother tells you that the baby is absolutely fine. She—the baby—seems awake, alert and active. You wonder if you imagined the sleep cues and decide to let the baby play for a while.

A few minutes later, the baby is yawning, frowning, asking for a feed, starting to get grumpy. Your mother has started rocking the baby to pacify her. You jump to action! You need a few minutes to settle down on a couch with your water, snacks, books and nursing pillow. By now, the baby is crying. When you try to nurse the baby, she's pulling away and fussing. When you try to rock her, she's arching her back and bawling. It takes you 30 minutes of vigorous rocking and chanting to get the baby to calm down, then nurse, and fall asleep.

So, what happened here? You were bang on target when you noticed the early sleep cues at the 30-minute awake window mark. When you went to the bathroom, your baby got overtired and her body released the stress hormone 'cortisol', giving her a shot of energy and a 'second wind' (see 'Overtiredness' in the Chapter 3, 'How to Get Your Baby to Sleep: The SHARED Method'). This is what made her seem alert and active to you again. A few minutes later, she started showing you late sleep cues. By the time you got settled to soothe her to sleep, she was grossly overtired, quite cantankerous and unable to fall asleep.

Even the most alert amongst us encounter this situation several times a week with babies because early sleep cues are so subtle and easy to miss. However, it is very important to watch for them every single time (be *'unagi'*, as Ross would say on *F.R.I.E.N.D.S.!*). Keep your baby's awake window in mind, prepare for sleep time in advance and be ready to pounce as soon as you see early sleep cues!

Circadian Rhythms

The approximately 24-hour cycle that runs our body processes in a timely, cyclical manner is called the circadian rhythm. The sleep–wake cycle is a part of this. While babies do receive the sleep hormone melatonin in the womb and from breastmilk, their day–night rhythm is weak and needs to form during their fourth trimester, normally between 2 and 3 months of age. Before this, babies often sleep at odd hours of the day and night. They usually do have a long stretch of sleep but it does not always align with our 'night'. In the first two months, babies are usually not affected by sound and light while they sleep. However, nor does it help to have lots of light during the day and darkness at night as they are not physiologically ready to develop an internal clock.

In the third month, however, it is important to keep babies in daylight from their morning wakeup until 6 p.m., then to keep them in a dim environment until bedtime and then make it pitch dark when they sleep. If the baby has started to get disturbed by light during daytime naps, it's okay to keep it dim or dark for the naps and then keep the baby in a lit environment while awake. Research has shown that 30 minutes of bright daylight in the first hour after wake-up can facilitate the setting of the circadian clock.

How does this sleep–wake pattern work? Light enters the eye and is detected at the retina. Information is relayed to the suprachiasmatic nucleus, which is the central clock in the brain that sends messages to other parts of the brain and body to trigger a flurry of activity. Melatonin, cortisol, body temperature, movement, blood pressure, digestion and consolidated sleep are all part of the circadian rhythm. For newborns, a rhythm of cortisol develops at 8 weeks of age, melatonin and sleep efficiency develop at approximately 9 weeks, and body temperature rhythm at 11 weeks.

Bedtime Routines

Babies may not know their nights from their days, but a solid bedtime routine helps from day one. A bedtime routine is a series of steps you take every day to signal bedtime is coming, like a gentle massage, changing into pyjamas, saying good night to objects and people around the house, reading a couple of books, singing lullabies. You can implement this at a fixed time every night, preferably close to the baby's long stretch of 'night sleep'. It is a time for your baby to unwind, to connect with you and to begin to understand that sleep time is coming.

The 4-Month Sleep Regression

Newborn sleep is mostly deep sleep. They drift between active and quiet sleep but there is no cyclical nature to these sleep stages, and the stages of quiet (or deep) sleep can be quite long. They also have a neurological stimulus barrier that prevents them from being greatly affected by sound and light. That is why babies sometimes sleep long stretches in the first few months. At 3½ months, most parents report that their babies are sleeping 5–7-hour stretches at night. We remember waking multiples times to check on our babies at that time because we couldn't believe they were sleeping such long stretches without any feeds! We would often wake up in the mornings in a pool of milk and thank our lucky stars for our miracle babies.

The miracle did not last, however, as, at around 4 months of age, baby sleep patterns undergo a massive change. Somewhere between 3 and 5 months, you may notice the following in your baby:

- Waking almost every hour at night to feed or be soothed
- More active night wakings
- Increased fussiness during naptimes and feeding sessions
- Short naps resulting in more crankiness
- Need for holding in arms throughout naps and frequent bridging of naps
- Sensitivity to sound and light while sleeping.

This bewildering and exhausting phase is the infamous 4-month sleep regression. There are several causes for it, including:

- Babies develop adult-like sleep cycles. That is, they start cycling through stages of light and deep sleep and wake at the end of each sleep cycle just like adults. But, unlike adults, they need help to fall asleep after each cycle. See Chapter 2, 'The Baby Superpower: Sleep' for information on sleep cycles.
- Babies become more aware of their surroundings and are consequently more easily stimulated and distracted.

A 'stimulus barrier' in their brains that previously prevented them from becoming overwhelmed no longer exists. This leads to overstimulation and overtiredness.

- Circadian rhythms have now formed and thus, the morning wake-up time starts drifting earlier. Parents need to assist to shift bedtime correspondingly earlier, which does not always happen.
- Babies drop their fifth nap, allowing bedtime to shift earlier, but requiring some management on the part of parents.
- Babies end up feeding less during the day as they are so easily distractible and so wake more at night to tank up.
- Mom's milk supply is no longer hormonally driven and so the baby needs to keep the supply up by waking more.

The 4-month sleep regression is one of the hardest phases of early parenthood. There is no way to entirely escape its effects, but we can try to ease it with a little bit of management. It's important to go with the flow without imposing a strict routine on our babies. We need to observe their cues and decide their subsequent sleep time based on how well they have slept at night or during the previous nap. Keeping a close eye for early sleep cues is very important as overtiredness is fuel for the regression. If the baby is highly stimulated and distracted, cues could be easy to miss, and so awake windows need to be kept in mind as well. Usually, 'awake windows or early sleep cues—whichever comes first' is a good rule to follow. Help your baby to drop the fifth nap by lengthening the previous four naps and shifting bedtime earlier.

It is also important to have a menu of ways to support their sleep—nursing, rocking, walking, babywearing, music, humming, shushing, alternative caregivers—all need to be kept at hand to be pulled out as needed! Be prepared to hold them for the entire duration of naps to preserve their sleep. Help in connecting or bridging their sleep cycles by staying close by and nursing or rocking back to sleep as soon as you see them stir awake. Start making it pitch dark and quiet for all naps and night sleep as babies now become easily distracted by stimuli.

The peak period of the regression lasts about two to three weeks, but since the development of sleep cycles is permanent, babies don't go back to sleeping long stretches as they did before the regression for quite a long time. Babies continue to wake frequently and need soothing. The ability to bridge sleep cycles independently develops slowly and is only fully developed by 2.5 to 3 years old.

Bridging of Naps

Since we now know that babies sleep in cycles, that they wake at the end of each sleep cycle and need help to start a new one, it follows that we need to be present with our babies to help them complete their sleep needs. Somehow, while we understand that our babies are waking at night and nursing or being rocked back to sleep, we often don't apply the same logic to naps. When they wake from a nap, we assume the nap is over and they are just up.

Babies waking up from a nap does not mean the nap is over. First and foremost, they wake at the end of a sleep cycle. However, they also wake because they are hungry or wet or hot or cold or have sensed separation or something has disturbed them, especially during their light sleep stages.

A slightly unromantic analogy for baby naps is the charging of a mobile phone. Every time your baby naps, your baby needs to recharge to 100 per cent like a phone. If your baby wakes up at 50 per cent charged, we need to plug the baby back in to sleep and ensure a full recharge.

At the newborn stage, babies usually need to be held in arms to ensure that they don't wake completely in the middle of a sleep cycle or when they are in light sleep. Sometimes, lying down next to them can work as well. When they wake, nursing, bottle-feeding or rocking can be used to soothe them back to sleep. It's a good idea to offer soothing every time the baby wakes as you don't know whether the baby has reached 100 per cent charge or not! An incomplete nap sets off a cycle of overtiredness and it is important to extend every nap to its optimal length.

Holding for Naps

Rasika had become a mom only a month before. Fortunately, most things were going well. The breastfeeding was off to a strong start. She felt she had understood how to rock and feed her baby Mia. She and her husband, Pramit, had got the hang of burping the baby, changing diapers, giving baths. There was one mysterious phenomenon, however, that had her pulling her hair out. Rasika or Pramit would soothe Mia to sleep by nursing or rocking. They would wait until the baby seemed to be in deep sleep. Then, very slowly and delicately, they would lower Mia into her cot. As soon as her body touched the mattress surface, baby Mia's eyes would pop open! And the whole process would begin again.

'Sometimes we manage to put her down in the cot or on our bed,' Rasika told us. 'But she still wakes 15–20 minutes later. The nap is never longer than that. We feel like we spend the whole day trying to get her to sleep and she still isn't sleeping enough!'

We told Rasika and Pramit to try one simple thing: to hold Mia in their arms for the entire duration of her naps. To just not put her down. At all. Two days later, Rasika reported that Mia was clocking 17 hours of sleep in the day. She was sleeping beautifully and was so much happier throughout the day!

So, what exactly happened here? What happened is that Rasika and Pramit gave baby Mia what her biological programming demanded—physical closeness and security while she slept. As we have discussed before, human babies are born at a very dependent stage of development and have a biological survival instinct that causes them to jerk awake if they sense separation from their caregiver while they sleep.

As Professor James McKenna says, 'Infants are biologically designed to sense that something dangerous has occurred—separation from the caregiver. They feel, through their skin, that something is different, such as missing the softness of the mother's touch, the heat of mother's body, the smell of mother's milk, the gentleness of the mother's moving, breathing chest and the feeling of being protected. Infants are alerted because, as far as their own body is concerned, they are about to be abandoned, and it is therefore time to awaken to call the caregiver back—the very caregiver on whose body the infant's survival depends.'

It is extremely common for babies to wake instantly when placed on a foreign surface or, if not instantly, as soon as they cycle into light sleep. This is particularly common with newborns but continues for most of the first year. By month 10 or 11, babies can usually be put down in a dark room, with a caregiver nearby. Some babies outgrow the need to be held earlier. Even after they outgrow the need, babies may need to be held during regressions or when they are ill or teething.

When we suggested this to Rasika and Pramit, their reaction was similar to that of most parents who hear this for the first time (and indeed what we also wondered while holding our babies for their naps initially): 'Won't this get my baby into the habit of always needing to sleep in someone's arms?'

There is no such risk. Babies do not form habits at this age. They have biological needs which change with time. A 3-month-old's needs are not the same as a 12-month-old's. Nothing that you do now is going to affect your baby's needs when they are older. The only thing that *will* happen if you don't hold your baby for naps is that you will have an overtired, sleep-deprived baby who is unhappy and much clingier when awake. The parenting mantra 'what you resist persists' definitely applies here. You can try to avoid holding, but you will suffer for it, and the need will not go away just because you are ignoring it.

See the Chapter 3, 'How to Get Your Baby to Sleep: The SHARED Method', for more tips and tricks linked to holding for naps.

6

Your Baby's Sleep: 5 to 7 Months

What Does Sleep Look Like Now?

Babies continue to feed and sleep often through the day. However, as their awareness grows, they are now easily distracted by their surroundings. Something as simple as a shadow on the wall or a crease in a curtain can captivate them completely, milk and sleep be hanged! Often, mothers of 5-month-olds complain that the baby doesn't feed sufficiently through the day, just snacking a few minutes at a time. This is due to their easy distractibility and the solution is to feed them in a dark and quiet room, possibly with some music playing to hold their interest.

By now, they are so easily stimulated by light and sound that they also need to sleep in quiet and dark rooms for both naps and nights. The happy-go-lucky newborn phase, when babies would sleep anywhere and everywhere, with the TV blaring, phones ringing and people talking, has come to an end. Now, the baby's naps are a designated time in the day when he needs to be taken to a dark and quiet room and sleep needs to be categorically facilitated.

Babies continue to wake easily when put down and therefore need holding in arms throughout naps. This carries on for many babies until 10–11 months of age though some may accept being placed on a bed by 5–6 months with a caregiver next to them. Some careful trial and error every two weeks lets us know if a baby is ready for this.

Babies' circadian rhythms have formed completely by the end of 4 months and so they start to wake earlier. They need a correspondingly early bedtime. They take four naps in a day from 5 to 6 months and then drop one nap and shift to a solid three-nap schedule.

They continue to wake regularly at night for both feeds and comfort. As we know, one of the key developments during the 4-month sleep regression is the emergence of sleep cycles. This is like an internal alarm clock for babies and many parents report that they could set their watches by how promptly their baby wakes at the end of 40 minutes! The development of sleep cycles means that babies need frequent bridging of sleep both for naps and at night.

Transition from Four Naps to Three

This is the first major nap transition you will be handling as a new parent and, we can assure you, it is not the last! The nap transitions that take place before this are somewhat blurry as sleep schedules can be fluid in the newborn stage. At the end of 5 months, however, your baby will clearly and categorically shift from taking four naps to taking three solid naps.

The basic architecture of every nap transition is:

- Awake windows increase
- Naps lengthen

- The number of naps reduces by one
- Bedtime shifts earlier.

Like with every nap transition, we as parents are tempted to jump the gun and drop the nap as soon as the early rumblings of the transition appear. These early rumblings, which will start to show up in the middle of the fifth month, are (i) resistance to the last nap and (ii) active night wakings. However, dropping the nap after a couple of days of resistance is a recipe for overtiredness. We need to find the sweet spot when our babies can stay awake for longer stretches without getting tired and are taking long enough naps earlier in the day to make it possible for the last nap of the day to seamlessly blend into bedtime.

The signs that your baby is absolutely ready to drop the nap will appear almost bang on the 6-month mark and will include some combination of:

- Nap resistance
- Bedtime resistance
- Short naps
- Early morning wakings
- Active night wakings.

Take care, though, that these signs should only be observed to indicate a nap transition if everything else is in place—like an age-appropriate schedule, proper sleep environment, physical closeness and the bridging of naps. If you are doing all of this and the baby is still showing the above symptoms, it is probably time to drop the fourth nap.

The way to drop the nap is to help the baby stay awake for slightly longer stretches and to facilitate slightly longer naps.

Here are some sample schedules to indicate how a nap transition may occur:

	5 Months	5.5 Months	6 Months
Wake up	7 a.m.	7 a.m.	7 a.m.
Nap 1	8–8.45 a.m.	8.15–9 a.m.	8.30–9.15 a.m.
Nap 2	10.15–11.15 a.m.	10.45–11.45 a.m.	11.15 a.m.–12.30 p.m.
Nap 3	1.15–3.15 p.m.	1.30–3.30 p.m.	3–5 p.m.
Nap 4	5.30–6.15 p.m.	6–6.30 p.m.	–
Bedtime	8.30 p.m.	9 p.m.	7.45 p.m.

As you can see, the transition is happening gradually over the whole month. The last two weeks will become quite tumultuous, with four naps on some days and three naps on others. It will probably take 2–3 weeks to settle down entirely and then your baby will be on a glorious, solid, 3-nap schedule!

6-Month Growth Spurt

Growth spurts are linked to physical or mental growth and feature increased feeding and some long sleep sessions. You may find that your baby is nursing round the clock, waking frequently to nurse at night or remaining latched for hours while sleeping. You may also find that your baby is taking some inordinately long naps, though with a fair amount of bridging. The baby may also be more fussy or clingy. Sometimes parents get tempted to introduce supplementary feeds at this point—either expressed breast milk or formula or solid food—but this is not a good idea as the baby increases your breastmilk supply by feeding more. The best way to handle them is to nurse on demand, hydrate yourself and eat well. Hold your baby as much as needed. At the 6-month mark, the growth spurt is usually linked to physical growth and a flurry of developmental milestones. Like all growth spurts, it passes in about 3–5 days.

Nursing to Sleep

At around this point in our parenting journey, we start wondering whether (or others around us start suggesting that) we are creating a bad habit or a bad sleep association by nursing our babies to sleep.

'Your baby is using you as a pacifier.'

'If you don't break this habit, your baby will never sleep well.'

'Your baby is waking so frequently because you are still breastfeeding.'

'If you allow your baby to fall asleep at the breast, your baby will wake expecting to still be at the breast.'

Any of these sound familiar?

In fact, every single one of these statements is incorrect. Nursing to sleep is the biological norm. It is how nature intended babies to sleep. The suckling motion promotes sleep and produces sleep hormones in both the mother and the baby. Breastmilk produced at night contains the sleep hormone melatonin which plays a vital role in regulating the baby's circadian rhythms. Babies also feed well when they are asleep, while they may be distracted when awake.

Moreover, nursing creates comfort and security. The physical closeness with the parent helps them sleep better. So, nursing is a perfectly designed sleep solution!

It's important to remember that babies do not form habits. Nor do they manipulate or 'remember' that they should do something to get a particular result. Their neocortex (thinking brain) is simply not developed enough. They only follow their biological programming and, when they can outgrow it naturally, they do.

If need be, nursing to sleep can be replaced by rocking or walking, especially with an alternate caregiver. This association can be created gradually over time, and most babies respond very well to multiple methods of falling asleep. Having said that, for the mom, nothing is easier and more convenient than nursing to sleep! It is much less labour intensive than rocking or walking or bottle-feeding. A mum can bedshare and nurse lying down. She barely needs to wake when her baby does. So, nursing to sleep leads to much more undisturbed and continual sleep for a mom.

Nursing is not only the easiest way to make our babies fall asleep, it is also the easiest way to bridge naps. When your baby wakes in the middle of a nap, a quick suckle can make them fall right back to sleep. In fact, whenever your baby wakes from a nap, we recommend that you offer a 'wake up feed'. This gives your baby the option of falling back asleep if she needs to. Even if her sleep is over or you feel she just nursed 20 minutes ago to bridge her nap, you should offer. She will most likely accept the feed. It will satiate her and give her a good start for her next awake window. She is now fuelled and ready to go—well-rested and well-fed—for a fair while!

Nursing is an invaluable sleep tool, apart from its many health benefits and parenting uses. And while it is natural, it is also a learned skill. If you are struggling with breastfeeding, seek help! There are so many wonderful resources, like the Facebook group *Breastfeeding Support for Indian Mothers*, books like *The Womanly Art of Breastfeeding* by the La Leche League or *Breastfeeding Made Easy* by Carlos González, your local La Leche League Leader or a qualified lactation consultant (preferably an International Board Certified Lactation Consultant).

Box 6.1 Bottle-Feeding Aversion

Babies who are primarily bottle-fed sometimes exhibit a puzzling behaviour that is now increasingly recognized as 'bottle aversion'. They are visibly distressed when they see their bottle of infant formula or breastmilk or sometimes even before, when they are placed in a feeding position or their bib is put on. They may resist feeding at all times when awake and accept their feeds only when asleep. The fact that your baby does feed when asleep helps to rule out a physiological obstacle to feeding. The aversion is a psychological or emotional response and is usually rooted in the baby having been force-fed at some point. This could be a single highly traumatic event or repeated exposure to feeding experiences that are unpleasant, stressful or painful. This could be the result of varying degrees of pressure, ranging from coercion to 'encouragement'. Often, parents who are concerned about their baby consuming a fixed amount of milk or gaining a certain amount of weight are anxious about how much their baby is feeding and can become insistent about the baby consuming more than the baby really wants to. A bottle-feeding aversion can definitely cause sleep disturbances because the baby will not fall asleep easily while hungry and yet will feed only when asleep. The solution to this situation is to expose the baby repeatedly to pleasant feeding experiences, where the baby is entirely in charge and absolutely no encouragement or force is used. Australian nurse Rowena Bennett puts forward a program in her book *Your Baby's Bottle-Feeding Aversion: Reasons and Solutions* where parents consciously work on rebuilding their baby's trust in them where feeds are concerned. We recommend using the programme outlined in this book and its related Facebook group and website to work through this issue, if you are facing it.

Introducing Solid Food

Babies are to be exclusively breastfed or formula-fed for the first 6 months of their life, according to recommendations by the WHO, UNICEF, the Indian Ministry of Health, the American Academy of Pediatrics (AAP), Health Canada and the Australian Department of Health. Babies are introduced to solid food after they turn 6 months old, when they exhibit developmental signs of readiness including sitting upright (with support, if needed), loss of the tongue-thrust reflex and an interest in food when they see people eating around them. At this point, some parents expect sleep to miraculously improve. This is an extension of the premise that babies wake because they are hungry, which we know to be misguided as babies wake for any number of reasons, the primary of which is sleep cycles. Therefore, feeding your baby solid foods is not going to make them sleep longer. A corollary to this is that one should not introduce solid foods earlier than recommended in the hope that this will help your baby sleep longer. In fact, sleep patterns become disrupted for 2–3 weeks after the introduction of solids due to massive changes in the digestive system, introduction of fibre and alterations in the bowel microflora. Even once that settles, babies usually continue to wake just as much as they did before and that is normal. The primary source of nutrition until the age of 1 year is breastmilk or formula; therefore, not only should the introduction of solid food be slow and preferably baby-led, it should not be expected to have a dramatic impact on anything, including sleep. It is important to not go overboard with solid food and to maintain a careful rhythm between milk, sleep and solids. After your baby wakes from a nap, nurse her. Offering solids without first offering milk can lead to milk being replaced disproportionately. Offer solids 45 minutes after the nursing session, by when the baby will have built up a bit of an appetite again. Allow the baby to decide what and how much to eat. Do not stress if the baby eats nothing or just a few bites. Many babies show no interest in food until they are 12, 13, even 14 months old. Once the baby is done with the meal—whether she has had 1 bite or 10 bites—offer to nurse again. Many breastfed babies eat as much as interests them but not to their hunger and then top up the meal with their favourite dessert: breastmilk. Do not skip nursing at bedtime even if you feel your baby has had a hearty dinner.

Parents often ask us if they can feed their babies something specific to aid in better sleep. Nothing that you feed your baby is going to have a transformative or even very significant effect on his sleep. Yes, some foods support sleep-inducing neurotransmitters such as serotonin and melatonin. These foods are rich in tryptophan and Vitamin B and are usually found in chicken, turkey, nuts, bananas and eggs. Foods rich in zinc, magnesium and essential fatty acids also help in the production of sleep and relaxation neurotransmitters.

Some anti-sleep foods should be avoided, especially in the second half of the day. These include sugar, coffee, chocolate, spicy food and gassy food. Presumably, your baby is not being introduced to much of this within the first year. Caffeine in a breastfeeding mum's diet could impact sleep. She should limit her intake to 2 cups per day but observe if even that much is affecting her baby's sleep. Although most babies do fine with a low level of caffeine in the mother's milk supply, some rare babies react quite strongly to even a bit of caffeine, especially in the early months. Sugar too is a stimulant and you may want to avoid even natural sugars in the second half of the day. Chocolate contains theobromine, which can negatively affect sleep. It can also be helpful to steer clear of 'gassy' foods such as broccoli, fried food and beans in the evening (both for the baby and the nursing mother). They may also disturb sleep by irritating the digestive system.

Thinking about Sleep Training?

Most sleep trainers and even old-school medical organizations and doctors advise sleep training babies (teaching them to 'self-soothe' by withholding comfort and causing distress) after the age of 4 or 6 months. In case you encounter this misinformation somewhere, please ignore it. See the chapter 'The Sleep Training Trap and the Myth of Self-Soothing' to understand why we do not recommend sleep training.

Bedtime Routine

Although a bedtime routine is valuable from a baby's very first day, it becomes quite important after a baby's circadian rhythms have formed and sleep patterns become more consistent. A bedtime routine is a series of steps that you take every night just before your baby's final sleep time to indicate that night sleep is coming. It could start with a bath or a sponge, a moist or dry massage, changing the diaper and putting on pyjamas, saying good night to objects and people around the house, going into a dim bedroom, reading some books, singing some lullabies, cuddling on the bed and then, finally, turning out the lights and feeding or rocking to sleep. A bedtime routine primes the baby mentally and physically to unwind and go to sleep. It is also a wonderful time of connection and bonding between the parent and the baby. This is an element of your routine that will stand you in good stead in the tumultuous toddler and pre-schooler days.

Should Your Baby's Schedule Adapt to the Family's?

Your baby now has a routine of his own and also the need for a particular sleep environment. This can sometimes come into conflict with the family's schedule. A parent or grandparent may be returning home late and an early bedtime may make it difficult for them to meet the baby. It may become difficult to make it to social commitments as the baby needs to sleep after a particular awake window and in a dark, quiet room, with a parent nearby for comfort and bridging.

What should you do in this situation? As far as possible, put the baby's needs first as the baby's needs are biological. Keeping a baby awake past her awake window or allowing her nap to get disrupted is just going to set off a vicious cycle of overtiredness. Family members who return late can spend time with their baby in the mornings. Social commitments can, as far as possible, be shifted to fit in the awake windows or, if the baby responds well, she can sleep in an ergonomic baby carrier. Your baby's sleep is intricately bound to her internal biological rhythms and is much less flexible than our adult lives. It will be more harmonious for everyone involved if the baby is allowed to follow that rhythm.

The Magic Cloak of Darkness

Since a baby's circadian rhythms form by months 3 and 4, there is no need to keep the baby in lit rooms during daytime naps.

As babies become more aware of their surroundings, they become very easily stimulated by seeing things around them and by the slightest sounds. Once babies turn 4–5 months old, it is a good idea to start making babies nap in a dark and quiet room. Even low visibility when they are being soothed to sleep or when they wake between sleep cycles or drift into light sleep can be very distracting for babies and cause them to fight sleep. Making the room pitch dark can give almost magical results—with babies falling asleep faster, waking less and falling *back* asleep after wakings more easily, leading to timely naps that are longer and easier to manage. Night lamps should also be avoided at night for the same reasons and the additional reason that any form of light obstructs the production of melatonin, the sleep hormone.

Soumya saw the effects of this magic trick for herself when her baby was 7 months old and she came to Himani for professional advice. Himani explained to her all the steps she needed to take—observe early sleep cues, follow awake windows and the recommended nap schedule for the baby's age, hold the baby for naps and bridge naps and, finally, ensure it is pitch dark for both daytime naps and night sleep. Soumya began to implement the recommendations. Her baby's sleep improved immediately when she instituted three naps totalling 4 hours of sleep with the correct awake windows and the correct length of night sleep. However, she was still struggling to extend naps. She would need to hold the baby for all naps, the baby took a very long time to fall asleep and bridging was hit and miss. The baby still seemed overtired throughout the day. When Himani went through the checklist of recommendations with her, everything seemed in place. Finally, Himani asked to do a video call to see the sleep environment for herself. Lo and behold! Soumya had religiously switched off all the lights and drawn the curtains for the daytime naps but, since light leaked from under and around the curtains, there was a fair amount of visibility in the room. It was enough to stimulate and distract the baby. Soumya was also still using a night lamp at night as she felt nervous about not being able to see her baby. Himani told her to stick black chart paper on the windows and to extinguish the night light. She explained to Soumya the pitch darkness test: can you see your hand in front of your face? If yes, it is not dark enough. Soumya ordered the black chart paper and went about blackening the room the next day. That very day, the naps were transformed! The baby fell asleep within minutes. Soumya did not have to hold her baby for any naps except the tricky third catnap. Naps were bridged easily by nursing in the side-lying position. They were beautifully long and restful. At night, she switched off the nightlight as well and used her mobile phone's screen to check on her baby whenever she woke and felt the need. The improved, restorative naps and the pitch darkness at night reduced the night wakings as well. Soumya had been sceptical about how much difference this one change could make, but the proof was in the pudding! The magic cloak of darkness had done its work.

Making a room pitch dark can seem a bit impractical, extreme, even annoying. However, it is usually non-negotiable for baby sleep. Even if you do everything else right, this one missing ingredient can make baby sleep an exercise in frustration for you. In fact, 100 per cent of the parents who have come to Himani for professional counselling have seen an immediate and dramatic improvement as soon as they have implemented this one recommendation diligently.

See the Chapter 3, 'How to Get Your Baby to Sleep: The SHARED Method', for some frequently asked questions on dark and quiet rooms.

What If the Mother Is Returning to Professional Work?

With most organizations in India offering 6 months of maternity leave, this is often the phase when mums return to professional work within or outside the home. This does not have to mean the end of biologically normal, baby-led sleep. It is possible to maintain your baby's routine, meet your baby's needs and have a well-rested, happy sleeper even if the mother is unavailable for a part of the day. See Chapter 10, 'Sleep for the Modern Parent: How to Handle Family Dynamics and Solo Parenting' for our discussion on this.

7

Your Baby's Sleep: 8 to 15 Months

What Does Sleep Look Like Now?

Babies transition from three naps to two naps between months 8 and 9 and continue to take two naps until sometime between 15 and 21 months. They follow the 2–3–4 pattern, which is often referred to as the 'golden period' of baby sleep! Their two naps total 3.5 to 4 hours of sleep and they sleep around 11 hours at night.

They continue to need physical closeness to their caregiver while sleeping. Many babies still wake when put down on the bed, though this usually fades away by 10–11 months at the latest, barring regression and teething phases. Even once they can be put down, babies need the warmth of a caregiver next to them and most certainly need bridging of their sleep cycles for both naps and night sleep. They do wake three to four times a night on average for both milk and comfort.

Babies are easily stimulated by light and sound at this age and continue to need a pitch dark and quiet environment to sleep in during the day or night. They do still need active forms of soothing like nursing, suckling on a bottle or rocking in arms. They experience acute separation anxiety and can call out vehemently for their primary caregiver. Packed with milestones, this period sees sleep regressions at 8–10 months and then again at 12 months.

The Transition from Three Naps to Two

This takes place once the baby is 8 or 9 months old (seldom before 8 months) and can take two to three weeks to be complete. Here are some signs that your baby may be ready for the transition:

- The baby is resisting naps.
- The baby is taking short naps.
- The baby is resisting bedtime.
- The baby is waking very early in the mornings.
- The baby is having active night wakings.

If you see some of these signs despite an age-appropriate sleep schedule, best attempts to bridge sleep and a pitch dark and quiet sleep environment, you may have a nap transition on your hands!

Please do not rush the transition. Expand the awake windows gradually until both the third nap and bedtime become quite late. Eventually, there will be no time left for the third nap and it will need to be dropped, with bedtime moving dramatically early to compensate.

Once the transition is complete, the baby will be on an elegant 2–3–4 pattern.

	3 Naps	2 Naps: Stage 1	Final 2–3–4 Pattern
Wake up	7 a.m.	6.30 a.m.	7 a.m.
Nap 1	8.45–9.45 a.m.	8.30–10.15 a.m.	9.00–11.00 a.m.
Nap 2	12 noon–1.30 p.m.	1.00–3.00 p.m.	2.00–4.00 p.m.
Nap 3	4.00–5.30 p.m.	–	–
Bedtime	8.30 p.m.	6.30 p.m. (temporary early bedtime)	8.00 p.m.

Box 7.1 The 2–3–4 Pattern

Start the first nap 2 hours after the baby wakes in the morning, the second nap 3 hours after the baby wakes from the first nap and night-time sleep 4 hours after the baby wakes from the second nap. The total of the two naps should be 4 hours. (If one of the naps is less than 1 hour long, the baby may not stay awake for all of the next awake window and will need to be taken to sleep earlier.)

The baby may expand these awake windows after 11–12 months, moving towards 2 hours 15 minutes—3 hours 15 minutes—4 hours 15 minutes.

8–10-Month Sleep Regression

This period in a baby's life sees many milestones and advancements. Babies undergo massive physical development, starting to crawl, pulling up to stand and slowly even cruising and walking with support. They experience huge cognitive leaps and brain development like word association, babbling, understanding cause and effect, being able to see across the room and responding to emotions like sadness and happiness. With so many exciting things happening, babies like to practise their new skills as much as they can, often in the middle of the night!

Babies now recognize familiar faces versus unfamiliar faces, leading to . . . *bingo!* stranger anxiety. They also understand object permanence—the idea that something they cannot see doesn't just disappear but *goes somewhere else*. This means that if Mumma goes out of the room, she exists somewhere else and needs to be called back! Hello, separation anxiety!

Add to this the fact that they are transitioning from three to two naps, sprouting quite a few teeth and becoming increasingly active, aware and over-stimulated—and we have a recipe for sleep regression!

Like with any regression, we need to ride it out. How can we ease it? See the Chapter 4, 'What Baby Sleep Looks Like: The Sleep Pyramid' for some tips and ideas on sleep regressions in general. For this one, in particular, be very mindful of holding the baby for naps and bridging sleep cycles, keeping it pitch dark and quiet for all daytime and night-time sleep and avoiding overtiredness at all cost. Help your baby to transition to two naps as that usually spells the end of the regression, but do not rush it as then you may have an overtired baby on your hands who is bound to be awake for long stretches in the middle of the night!

12-Month Sleep Regression

Just as you get a breather from the 8–10-month regression, you may find yourself dealing with yet another regression, this time linked to the walking milestone. Babies tend to resist naps majorly during this regression, leading parents to believe that their baby wants to move to a single nap from two naps. However, this is a false alarm. Babies do continue to need two naps until somewhere between 15 and 21 months. As they start walking, they also get tired more frequently and need those period breaks in the day.

Instead of dropping a nap, try expanding your baby's awake windows. From 2–3–4, you can move to 2.5–3.5–4.5 or something less symmetrical. Here is a simple formula that can help you figure it out:

- If your baby is taking a long time to fall asleep (more than 20 minutes) with lots of protesting/playing but then still takes a good nap (over 1 hour 15 minutes) that she wakes up happy from, try starting that nap 15 minutes *later*.
- If your baby falls asleep quickly at naptime, but then takes a short nap (under 1 hour) that he wakes up happy from, try starting that nap 15 minutes *later*.
- If your baby falls asleep quickly for a nap, but then takes a short nap (under 1 hour) that she wakes up crying from, try starting the nap 15 minutes *earlier*.
- If your baby falls asleep quickly for a nap and then takes a long nap (over 1.5 hours), you've found the sweet spot!

Keep in mind, though, that the above guidelines include the bridging of naps, a pitch dark room and active forms of soothing. The delay in naps or shortening of naps should be happening despite these things for you to conclude that you need to shift the nap. Otherwise, you need to first address these basics.

Is a Delayed Bedtime Okay?

In general, babies do well with an early bedtime as outlined in Chapter 3, 'How to Get Your Baby to Sleep: The SHARED Method'. However, during nap transitions, bedtime usually shifts later and that's okay. As awake windows expand, bedtime drifts later and later. Once the extra nap is dropped, bedtime shifts early again, until the same cycle repeats itself as the baby moves towards the next nap drop. However, what we call an early bedtime is 7 p.m. and a late bedtime is 10 p.m. If you are following your baby's biological rhythms as defined in this book, you will likely have a bedtime of between 7 and 8.30 p.m. for 70 per cent of baby- and toddlerhood, with a later bedtime for just a few pre-transition months.

The Expanding Awake Windows after the Baby's First Birthday

After the 12-month sleep regression, once you find yourself back on a steady two-nap routine, you will likely face ever-expanding awake windows and the aforementioned late bedtimes. This is expected and nothing to be alarmed about. Please do not drop to a single nap hastily. Most babies continue to take two naps until at least 15 months of age. You can allow awake windows to expand as per the formula shared earlier in the chapter and it may reach something like 3–4–5. This is usually the last stop on the train to One-Nap Land.

Do You Need to Wean from Breastfeeding?

As you approach your baby's first birthday, you may wonder if you need to wean from breastfeeding. Your elders or friends or even paediatrician may suggest that you have done it for long enough and now it is, at best, not of much value and, at worst, a bad habit you will never get rid of.

Well, we already know that nursing to sleep is not a bad habit and is, in fact, the biological norm. The WHO recommends breastfeeding for a minimum of 2 years. Anthropologist Katherine Dettwyler has argued that the natural age of weaning for human babies is between 3 and 5 years by looking at various 'life history' variables (such as the length of gestation, birth weight, growth rate, age at sexual maturity, age at the eruption of teeth, life span, etc.) in primates and correlating them with their age of weaning, then extrapolating that to humans.

Breastmilk also continues to provide nutrition and antibodies in the second year of life and beyond. According to Kathryn G. Dewey, in the second year (12–23 months), 448 ml of breastmilk provides

- 29 per cent of energy requirements
- 43 per cent of protein requirements
- 36 per cent of calcium requirements
- 75 per cent of vitamin A requirements
- 76 per cent of folate requirements
- 94 per cent of vitamin B12 requirements
- 60 per cent of vitamin C requirements.

So, it is not only biologically normal and healthy to continue breastfeeding well past the first year, but also extremely difficult to wean gently as one is fighting against something that comes naturally to babies. We would go so far as to say that if a baby has a deep nursing relationship with you, it is almost impossible to wean without tears before the age of 3 years and without a process that borders on the kind of harmful sleep training that we advise against. If at all you need to wean, it would need to be done very gradually over several months and with a lot of help from another caregiver.

Breastfeeding is an invaluable sleep tool and can see you through regressions, teething, illness and regular wakings with minimal fuss. It is also a wonderful parenting tool in general and can be a source of connection, emotional regulation, comfort and so much more in your relationship with your child. In general, the benefits of breastfeeding to natural term—or when the baby weans naturally—far outweigh the costs, if any.

Box 7.2 Does Breastfeeding at Night Cause Dental Caries?

You may have heard the common myth that breastfeeding at night once your baby has teeth can lead to dental caries. This is an extension of the basic oral health rule that babies (and older children and adults) should not consume anything after brushing their teeth at night. But there is no evidence that breastmilk causes tooth decay though, of course, breastfed babies should also maintain good dental hygiene in general. Breastmilk that is consumed straight from the source does not pool in the mouth like milk from bottles does. It also enters the mouth behind the teeth. Additionally, breastmilk contains lactoferrin, which fights the bacteria that cause tooth decay.

Do I Need to Wean the Bottle?

The AAP recommends weaning bottles by the age of 18 months. Some organizations recommend weaning at 12 months. This encompasses bottles containing all kinds of milk—human, animal or formula. Bottles do cause pooling of milk in the mouth and can cause tooth decay if used at night. Bottles can also cause dental issues like overbite or tooth protrusion. They have been linked with respiratory risks as well. However, weaning bottles needs to be approached with a lot of care and empathy. As we know, children do have a suckling instinct which they naturally outgrow sometime between 3 and 7 years. Breastfed babies do not need to be deprived of it but bottle-fed babies do, which is immensely unfair to the babies. Therefore, bottle-weaning should not be harsh or abrupt. It should be done over several months with a progressive transition to cups. Milk consumed at night from a bottle can be diluted with water very, very gradually—like 10 ml every two weeks—so that the baby's body gets used to taking in those calories during the day and accustomed to consuming water instead of milk at night.

Box 7.3 Hot Tip: Use a Video Baby Monitor!

This has been Himani's most prized baby-related possession! A video baby monitor is a nifty device that allows you to watch your sleeping baby from outside the room. You can leave your baby in a pitch dark and quiet room and yet dash back inside as soon as he stirs and you need to bridge sleep or soothe or comfort. You don't need to leave a door open and allow light or sound to leak in. You don't need to wait for your baby to wake up to the extent that they cry or call out. And you don't need to stay inside with them throughout if you don't want to.

The video baby monitor allows you to step out after bedtime (once the baby is in deep sleep, often after a long spell of cluster feeding while asleep), eat your dinner, finish work, watch TV, spend time with your partner, have some me-time without compromising or risking your baby's sleep in the slightest. You can pop back in to nurse or soothe them as needed and then pop back out again. Once your baby no longer needs to be held for naps, the video monitor will become your best friend during the day as well.

8

Your Baby's Sleep: 16 Months to 3 Years

What Does Sleep Look Like Now?

Babies transition from two naps to one somewhere between 15 and 21 months and continue to take that single nap until somewhere between 3 and 5 years. As you can see, there is a vast range within which these transitions occur. As babies grow older, the range for transitions increases. Of course, this means that things are a bit trickier for parents and there are longer rocky periods as well. That is part and parcel of toddlerhood!

A wise mother once said: 'If you thought infant sleep was hard, toddler sleep will kick your teeth in!' Toddler sleep is indeed a completely different ball game from infant sleep. While the latter is driven almost entirely by biological rhythms and fairly simple mathematics, sleep after the age of 1 year takes on a new dimension—that of behaviour and personality. It is normal for toddlers to push boundaries, test limits and assert their individuality in all spheres of their life, including sleep. Their activity levels are so high that it becomes increasingly difficult to identify sleep cues and also wind them down for sleep.

The immense speech and cognitive development they undergo do not help either, punctuating this period with several sleep regressions, most notably at 16, 18, 21 and 24 months. They are now more aware than ever and separation anxiety is at its peak.

And yet, toddlers are still little babies. While they can usually be put down on beds to sleep for their naps (except during certain phases like teething and regressions, when they may need holding in arms again), they do still need physical closeness with a caregiver in the form of lying next to them or periodic patting and rocking. They continue to need an active form of soothing to sleep, like nursing or rocking or walking. They continue to be easily stimulated by light and sound. It is normal for them to wake often at night—three to four times on average but as much as five to eight times during teething and regression phases.

Toddler Sleep Cues

Early	Late
• Rubbing eyes	• Hyperactivity
• Pulling hair	• Yawning
• Clumsiness	• Tantrums
• Fussiness with food	• Burying head in your chest
• General slowing down	• Fussiness and crankiness
• Lack of engagement	• Resistance to going to bed
• Jerky movements	• Asking for bed
• Losing interest in toys	• Grizzling
Some of the early cues could really be late cues. It depends on the degree. With time and a little trial and error, you'll probably be able to read your own toddler's cues quite clearly.	

Transition to One Nap

Babies start transitioning to one nap between 15 and 21 months. This is a lengthy process and one can often feel the rumblings as early as 13–14 months. It is important, however, to not rush the transition and support our babies to continue taking two naps as long as possible to avoid overtiredness and unnecessary stress on their systems. The transition itself can also take up to 2 months to stabilize.

We mentioned when discussing the 12-month sleep regression that parents often mistake it to be the transition to one nap. This is a false alarm and babies usually come back to taking two solid naps in a few days. It helps to expand awake windows a bit.

This process of expanding awake windows continues for a while. By the age of 15 months, babies are often following a 3–4–5 pattern, with the first nap starting 3 hours after the morning wakeup, the second nap 4 hours after the end of the first nap and bedtime 5 hours after waking from the second nap. The two naps continue to total about 3.5 hours of sleep. With such large awake windows, bedtime can be expected to be late and night sleep to total not more than 10 hours. This is a temporary phase and bedtime shifts early again once babies drop the second nap.

As the gaps before and between naps increase steadily, the morning nap becomes the single nap of the day and the afternoon nap dissolves into bedtime. Parents can help by allowing the gaps to increase. So, the gap before the first nap may increase from 2 hours to 3–3.5 hours. Then the gap between the first and second naps may increase from 3 to 4–4.5 hours. This will not happen in one day but in increments of 15 minutes every few days. The increased gap will ensure that the baby falls asleep easily and stays asleep longer.

There is a long phase when the baby still needs two naps but her ability to stay awake is lengthening. Her bedtime may start taking place 5 hours after waking from the second nap. In a case where a baby's normal bedtime used to be 7.30 p.m., once the second nap starts taking place post 4 p.m. and bedtime hits 10 p.m., it is time to drop the second nap and move to a super early bedtime of 5.30 or 6 p.m. Over time, this will drift back to her usual 7.30 p.m. For a long time, the single nap will happen quite early in the day and may not always be long enough.

The critical element in this transition is helping the baby to lengthen (i) the gap before the first nap and (ii) the duration of the first nap itself. It is only once the first nap is starting 3.5 hours after the morning wake–up and is at least 2.5 hours long that we can drop the second nap and go straight to bedtime.

In the initial single-nap phase, the nap may occur 3.5 hours after the baby wakes in the morning and be 2.5 hours long, with bedtime 5.5 hours after it ends. So, say, the baby wakes up at 6.30 a.m. Her nap would be from 10 a.m. to 12.30 p.m. She would need to be put to bed at 6 p.m. Then, over the months, the first gap will become 4 hours long and the second gap around 6 hours.

Sample schedules:

	2 Naps	1 Nap Transition	1 Nap Final
Wake up	6.30 a.m.	6.30 a.m.	6.30 a.m.
Nap 1	10.00–11.45 a.m.	10.15 a.m.– 12.45 p.m.	10.30 a.m.– 1.30 p.m.
Nap 2	3.15–5.00 p.m.	–	–
Bedtime	10.00 p.m.	6.30 p.m. (possibility of an active night waking)	7.30 p.m.

16-, 18-, 21- and 24-Month Sleep Regressions

To complicate matters further, babies undergo sleep regressions regularly in this period linked to an explosion of language and cognition in the second half of the second year.

Some signs of these regressions are:

1. The baby being overtired but resisting sleep due to the fear of missing out while she sleeps.
2. Not being able to sustain the entire day on one nap.
3. Separation anxiety.
4. Teething.
5. Testing limits and experimenting for the sake of it ('what happens if I do this?' behaviour).
6. Active night wakings and early morning wakings.

The first three regressions coincide with the transition to one nap. Parents of babies who are still on two naps might mistake this for the transition but find that the baby reverts to two naps in a few days. Parents of babies who have already transitioned to one nap may find that the baby is sleeping poorly at night or waking early in the morning or resisting naps or bedtime and, as a result of all this, not getting enough sleep and needing two naps. Again, the baby will revert to one nap after a few days.

Like with all regressions, we need to go with the flow without imposing a routine while ensuring that we avoid overtiredness to the maximum extent possible. We need to help in bridging early morning sleep and naps. Bedtime should be moved early if naps are too short. It helps to have a solid and lengthy bedtime routine to help toddlers unwind for the night.

After the 24-month sleep regression, toddlers usually have a fairly smooth one nap schedule, with slightly increased awake windows of 4.5 hours and 6.5 hours for most of the year after their second birthday.

Box 8.1 Hot Tip: When to Serve Lunch

Most of us assume that lunch should be served before a single nap. This is linked to the idea that babies sleep better after heavy meals and that naps should happen in the middle of the day. However, we recommend serving lunch *after* the single nap because the 4-hour awake window before the nap is too short a gap for breakfast, a snack *and* lunch. The longer 6-hour gap in the second half of the day allows for a well-spaced lunch, snack and dinner. If your baby wakes at 7 a.m. and naps from 11 a.m. to 2 p.m., lunch cannot be served before the nap at 10 a.m. It will have to be at 3 p.m. itself and, though that seems late by adult standards, babies do not read clocks in the same way or follow manmade labels for their meals. They are perfectly comfortable with this routine where they still get their three meals and two snacks on time.

Box 8.2 My Baby Takes Short Naps!

We regularly encounter sleep scenarios where a toddler is either taking two naps long past the recommended age or is overtired and cranky with a single nap or is having active wakings with a single nap. All of these scenarios are linked with the single nap (or the first nap) being too short. It is essential for the single nap of the day to be 2.5 to 3 hours long. This is not something a baby can achieve without support. Here is how you can ensure a long and restorative nap:

1. Follow the correct awake window before the nap so that the baby is not overtired.
2. Ensure that the room is pitch dark so that the baby falls asleep easily at the right time and also falls back asleep after bridging.
3. Stay with your baby during the nap and effectively bridge the nap.

Bedtime Battles

Prolonged bedtimes are a common feature of toddler sleep. Parents often come to us with complaints of toddlers being taken to bed at 9 p.m. and not sleeping before midnight. Toddlers do push boundaries and are often also so absorbed in their own universe that they can be difficult to push from Task A to Task B. However, there is definitely a lot that parents can look into where bedtime delays are concerned.

1. Rule Out Scheduling Issues
    Is your toddler taking two naps when she needs one? Is her single nap too short, leading to overtiredness and sleep resistance? Is the gap before the nap too long? Importantly, are we observing the 6 to 6.5-hours awake window after the single nap? Often, parents put their toddlers down for their naps after lunch and in the afternoons, say for 2–4 p.m., and then expect their toddlers to be down for the night by

8 or 9 p.m. As we know, the awake window after the single nap is 6 to 6.5 hours so a baby who is waking by 4 p.m. will not sleep before 10 or 10.30 p.m.

2. Manage the Second Half of the Day Suitably
    Ensure a little physical activity, preferably followed by a warm bath. Just as important as physical exercise, however, is art. Build some creative expression into their day because, as internationally renowned family counsellor Kim John Payne says, 'the creative process involves a letting go of conscious thoughts and ideas, and such opportunities for artistic release during the day help a child surrender into sleep'. Avoid sugar and chocolate in the evenings. Avoid screen time for at least two hours before bedtime as blue light from screens obstructs the production of melatonin.

3. Remove Sources of Light and Stimulation in the Room
    Is it pitch dark and quiet (apart from music, if any) once the bedtime routine is over and you are soothing your baby to sleep by nursing or rocking or walking? This final stage of soothing needs to be in pitch darkness to remove all stimulation or it will be extremely difficult for a toddler to fall asleep.

4. Manage Normal Toddler Limit Testing Behaviour
    Toddlers need a little managing, negotiation and coaxing throughout the day, whether it is concerning meals or changing their clothes or brushing their teeth or getting them out the door! Sleep time is no different. A little gameplay and coaxing and redirection are needed to get them through the bedroom door.

5. Address Any Fear, Anxiety or Stress in Their Lives
    Toddlers do feel fear and anxiety as a result of their
    experiences. It can help to validate their feelings and
    reassure them. Falling asleep involves a 'leap of faith', as
    Kim John Payne calls it. It requires trust and a feeling of
    connectedness. For this reason, we do recommend that the
    bedtime routine and final night soothing be done by the
    primary caregiver(s). It can help to ask the child simple
    questions about her day and help the child to 'unpack'
    difficult or distressing events of the day, interspersed with
    happy memories, while the parent simply listens and
    validates, without offering judgement or ready fixes. It
    can also help to share a little bit about what the child can
    expect the next day to look like. Payne suggests to do this
    with visuals (like pointing at the child's clothes laid out
    for the next day or offering the image of a tree the child
    will stand under outside school while waiting for parents
    to pick her up) as these visual markers are processed by the
    child while asleep. 'Whatever happens in those mysterious,
    healing processes of sleep, you can be sure that if your
    child has a concern, you'll hear about it the next morning,'
    says Payne.

6. Have a Solid Bedtime Routine
    At 16–18 months, serve dinner 1.5 hours before the
    intended sleep time. At 2 years, serve dinner 2 hours before.
    Have a lengthy, predictable and enjoyable bedtime routine
    after dinner that signals to your toddler to wind down
    and prepare for bed. Include calming activities like talking
    about their day, colouring and storytelling. Keep around 45
    minutes in mind for the final soothing, whether it is nursing

or rocking or walking. It is common for 'sleep onset latency' (or falling asleep) to take that long for toddlers.

7. Once Inside the Bedroom, the Baby Should Not Leave It
Toddlers have major FOMO and also no impulse control, which sometimes leads to them dashing out of the room when struck by an awesome idea about something that exists outside of it. This is to be avoided. Leaving the bedroom in the middle of the bedtime routine usually means a hard reset and having to start from scratch. The bedtime routine within the bedroom should be so consistent and enjoyable that the toddler is entirely absorbed and does not even think of leaving the room. If the baby is extremely insistent and only if the house outside the bedroom is dim and quiet as well, you could take her out for a few rounds of the living room. This can sometimes even help to break the cycle of bedtime delay. However, if there is activity outside the room, it is best to pre-empt this kind of insistence. Of course, if the baby gets flustered and cannot at all be redirected gently from this desire to leave, you might not have a choice. In that case, you'll need to agree to leave the room but also accept that tonight is a washout and you'll try again tomorrow.

8. Use an Active Method of Soothing
Toddlers usually cannot fall asleep simply lying down next to us before the age of 3.5 to 4 years. They are unable to keep still and wait for sleep to come. Expecting them to fall asleep just lying next to us is a recipe for delay and overtiredness as they will only become more and more stimulated as they wriggle about and keep trying to play on the bed. Toddlers need an active form of soothing like nursing, rocking or

walking. Even if we are able to bridge their sleep by cuddling after the age of 3 years, they usually need an active form of soothing at the time of falling asleep even at 4 years.

Is It Time to Wean Breastfeeding?

Sometimes, parents try to wean from breastfeeding at 18 months. Once they hit the WHO minimum recommendation of 2 years, they feel it would be safe to wean. However, they usually find that toddlers are not ready to give up nursing as yet and weaning can be extremely difficult.

It can come as a rude shock, therefore, that weaning even by the age of 3 years does not happen without tears and struggle. It is not necessary to wean from breastfeeding at this or, in fact, any stage. The natural age of weaning, as discussed before, is between 3 and 7 years. After the age of 3.5 or 4 years, even mother-led weaning is easier and often takes only a little nudge. It is our recommendation to acknowledge your child's resistance to weaning as a sign that he isn't ready and allow nature to take its course. Breastfeeding remains a wonderful source of nutrition and antibodies and an invaluable parenting and sleep tool.

Rishika Vipin Menon thought that she would end her breastfeeding journey when her daughter, Aathira, turned 6 months old and began to consume solids.

New mom, first time mom. Of course, I didn't know better!' she now chuckles. 'Fast forward 6 months into my breastfeeding journey; I realized that breastfeeding was a golden weapon that I could wield in any situation—hunger, thirst, boredom, tantrums, sickness, growth spurt but, most important of all, SLEEP. Nursing was the easiest and the quickest method to help my daughter fall and stay asleep.

I knew right then that I was going to hold on to my golden
weapon for as long as my daughter and I wanted.

Murmurs about weaning her daughter off breastfeeding began
within Rishika's family when Aathira turned 2 years old. 'When
the Covid lockdown began in April 2020, I succumbed to pressure
and tried to wean her night feeds cold turkey,' Rishika recalls. 'It
was a bad idea. My daughter was shocked to see that her safe place,
my breasts, were no longer accessible to her.' On the first day,
she took a little longer to sleep and asked to feed repeatedly but
managed to sleep eventually after countless stories. The little girl's
frustration turned to tears the second day. 'That was my breaking
point,' Rishika says. 'I knew that this was really not worth it. I let
her come back to nurse and she caressed my breasts like a mother
caresses her loving child and nursed to her heart's content.'

Rishika continued to talk to her daughter about cuddling
instead of nursing but did not actively try to wean her. She
understood that her baby was not ready. It was around the time
that Aathira was 3.5 years old that Rishika attempted to wean
again. She and her husband had just found out that they were
pregnant and her nipples felt overly sensitive. They had already
been speaking to her about weaning for many months and so,
one night, Rishika let her know that they would be hugging and
sleeping tonight. After many questions, little Aathira agreed.
'I realized through this experience that rushing into weaning
with force is not a good idea,' Rishika ruminates. 'Natural-
term weaning happens anytime between 3 and 7 years. Around
3.5 years, their maturity in terms of thinking jumps threefold.
It's easier on them when you explain yourself to them. No tears,
no frustration. We ended our breastfeeding journey on the right
note and the bond will stay with us forever.'

If you are wondering about weaning the bottle, see Chapter 7, 'Your Baby's Sleep: 8 to 15 Months'.

Night Weaning

As we have discussed in the previous chapter, breastmilk continues to hold significance in the second year of life as well. Night nursing can come to the rescue during such rough phases when your toddler needs more comforting, like during 18–24 months, when teething and speech development are at their peak and wakings become more frequent. Also, nursing can soothe teething pain and provide overall comfort that the child sorely requires at this time.

If you have been trying to wean during this phase, and it's proving difficult and leading to a lot of crying, it's because your child is going through a difficult and complex time and needs all the comforting he or she can get. If your toddler is resisting, it means she is not ready to wean. It's a good idea to wait and try again later, if you would still like to. The closer the baby is to self-weaning the easier it will be on both the baby and the parents, contrary to the popular belief that it is easier to wean while the baby is younger.

Types of Weaning

Weaning can happen in many ways: mother-led weaning (where the mother encourages the baby to drop feeds), child-led weaning (where the baby decides when to drop feeds), and partial weaning (where you drop some feeds, during the day or night). Often, we are aware of only the first option and not the other two. It is important to take an informed decision on weaning by being aware of the pros and cons of each of these options.

Feeling Pressured to Wean?

Many mothers feel the pressure to wean because of lack of support and misinformation about breastfeeding. Some mothers feel touched out and find themselves desperate to wean. Momentary aversion to breastfeeding, known as 'nursing aversion', is common and may be caused by hormonal imbalances or nutritional deficiencies. You do not need to live with this and can seek medical help. Aversion can also be caused by lack of rest and sleep. Temporary aversion is normal and natural and does not necessarily mean you need to wean. It can just be an indication that you need some help and a break from the overwhelming demands of parenting and feeding a baby. It is important to seek appropriate support and vent to someone close. Often, mothers find that getting adequate rest, assistance in childcare and a supportive spouse who shares nightwakings helps them continue their nursing journey well into toddlerhood. Many continue to nurse till the child self-weans, which is called natural or full-term weaning, and it can typically happen anytime between the ages of 2 and 5 years, sometimes beyond.

Busting Common Myths

There are many myths about breastfeeding and the need to wean a child early. Relatives, neighbours, well-meaning friends and even strangers do like to offer words of wisdom related to weaning but it's important to be able to separate fact from fiction. Before you consider weaning, please note some facts based on scientific research:

- Breastmilk has many benefits beyond 12 months.
- Weaning does not increase intake of solids and therefore the weight of the baby.
- Weaning at night will not guarantee that the baby sleeps through the night.
- Weaning will not necessarily ensure better sleep for the mother and baby and it is not a one-stop solution to exhaustion. Weaning often means you will need to employ more tedious ways of soothing the child to sleep such as walking and rocking.
- Your child will learn to sleep without nursing as he or she grows older, even if you do nothing to break the association.
- Some babies do sleep longer stretches post weaning but most do not and continue to wake up at night. This is because sleeping longer stretches has a strong link with brain maturity and your baby will be able to self-soothe once he is developmentally ready, which is typically around the age of 3–4 years.

How to Wean

If you are aware that weaning may not mean your baby will sleep longer stretches and if you still want to wean, then here are ways to make it less traumatic for the child and less stressful for you:

- It's best to take a gentle, gradual and flexible approach to weaning that is respectful towards both the needs of the mother and the child. Sudden weaning is not fair to the child. Please do not use neem paste or anything bitter on your nipples to turn a child off nursing as this can be traumatic too.

- You will need to find a new sleep association that is acceptable to the child, such as rocking/walking/patting/singing the baby back to sleep. You could feed the baby and then switch to any of these methods so the baby gets used to it.

- If the baby refuses any other form of comfort from the mother, you could feed the child and then hand him over to another caregiver who can soothe the child to sleep. Often, babies associate different modes of soothing with different caregivers so having an alternate caregiver around is very important when you are weaning. The father being involved is very helpful.

- Crying is not an inevitable part of weaning. Gentle and gradual weaning should involve no tears as the child's needs are being changed before they are being taken away. Weaning that involves crying can border on sleep training and should be avoided for the same reasons.

- Drop one feed at a time, not all together.

- Some toddlers understand and accept the concept of 'no dudu when it's dark outside' or 'you can have dudu once the sun comes up'. This typically works with older toddlers, aged 2–3 years. You could also look for children's books to read to your toddler about weaning or make your own book with your child.

- Many mothers report that day weaning toddlers is easier than night weaning so, if that is something that works for you, consider day weaning first, wait for some months, and then try night weaning.

- Weaning can take a few months when done gently and without letting the child cry. It's normal for a child to be more cranky and clingy and resist sleep while being weaned. Weaning requires patience and understanding.
- Weaning can be an emotionally exhausting process for the mother and baby and so it's important that both are ready for it. If the baby isn't ready to wean but the mother would like to, then a lot of extra cuddles and affection to replace the nursing will go a long way in making it less stressful for everyone.

How Can You Fit in Toddler Classes or Preschool?

Do try to fit any toddler classes around your baby's sleep schedule, instead of the other way round. See the Chapter 9, 'Your Baby's Sleep: 3 to 5 Years' for a more detailed discussion on this.

9

Your Baby's Sleep: 3 to 5 Years

What Does Sleep Look Like Now?

Toddlers continue to take one nap until sometime between 3 and 5 years of age. We mustn't rush this transition as surviving an entire day without a nap is very tough on little bodies. Dropping the last nap is a very slow process and can take 6–8 months. Bedtime may be delayed while they are still taking the nap and a bedtime between 9 and 10.30 p.m. is quite normal in such cases. After they drop the nap, the bedtime should shift to around 7 p.m.

Toddlers continue to need sleep cycles bridged for their naps and nights until somewhere between 3 and 4 years of age when they begin to bridge almost all their sleep cycles on their own. They may still wake for other reasons, like from a nightmare or out of anxiety, or because they are too hot or too cold or need to use the toilet or because something has disturbed them. However, the periodic waking at the end of a sleep cycle usually does fade away by this age.

At this age, the need for active forms of soothing—like nursing or walking them to sleep—may also slowly give way to more passive modes like lying next to them, cuddling them or patting them. They do, however, need a parent next to them to fall asleep and will likely look for a parent if and when they wake from sleep.

They continue to be easily stimulated by sound and light, though this too may ease at around 4 years of age. While we would still not recommend toddlers sleeping in bright daylight or with televisions on, they may be less easily disturbed by light from a phone screen or soft talking or doors clicking.

The last documented sleep regression is at 2 years, but babies do go through upheavals in their sleep regularly after that as well. Every few months, children go through massive cognitive and/or physical leaps, and sleep is inevitably disturbed at this time.

Children are still not inherently ready to shift to their own rooms and to sleep alone even at the end of this period. They still very much depend on the security and comfort of physical closeness to their parents in order to sleep well.

Dropping the Last Nap

If your child is between 3 and 5 years old (or older) and showing two or three of the following signs, the baby is likely ready to drop the final nap:

- The toddler's awake windows have expanded and bedtime is extremely late.
- The child resists the nap and/or resists bedtime even if awake windows, sleep environment and soothing method are optimal.
- The toddler takes a very short nap despite a pitch-dark room and despite our attempts to bridge the nap.

- The toddler has active night wakings or early morning wakings.
- The child starts clocking less than 11–11.5 hours of sleep in 24 hours.

Do try to hold on to the nap for as long as possible since making it through the day without a nap can be a lot of pressure on a little toddler's body. It can lead to overtiredness quite easily and it's likely that their night sleep will be disturbed. As we know, naps have a different function from night sleep. Not only do babies and toddlers need that recharge to not be overtired, but naps also have a developmental purpose and are vital for brain growth, attention spans and processing new learning. Neural connections are formed during sleep. Babies and toddlers who need a nap but are not offered one also behave very differently from well-rested babies. They may not eat well, and may be cranky, hyperactive and/or clumsier.

Now, *you* may understand the importance of the nap but, try as you may, your tot is just not taking the nap! Naps do require a little extra effort on the part of the caregiver during this transition phase. It is essential to have all the ingredients for a perfect nap, which are:

1. A pitch-dark, zero-stimulation room (it should be so dark that you can't see your hand).
2. Awake windows:
   At 2.5 years, it may be 4.5 hours before the nap and 6.5 hours between nap and bedtime. At 3 years, it may be closer to 5 hours and then 6.5 to 7 hours. The nap should be 2.5 to 3 hours long before the age of 3 years, after which it could dip to 2 hours on some days.

So, the nap needs to be early enough in the day or bedtime will be inordinately delayed. The baby should not be woken from the nap or in the mornings.

3. Pre-nap routine: a relaxing and enjoyable set of two or three activities that take place in the nap room, like reading books, colouring, doing puzzles or cuddling with the parent.

4. Active soothing method: tots do need nursing or walking until around 3.5 to 4 years of age, after which lying down and cuddling them may work.

5. Music with the soothing method: Music absorbs and focuses their active minds as you nurse or walk or cuddle them, allowing them to drift off.

If even one of these ingredients is missing, the nap won't happen.

It's important to keep in mind that it usually does take 30 minutes of active soothing for babies to fall asleep for the nap and 1 hour for bedtime. So, an ideal schedule at 2 to 2.5 years would be:

7 a.m.	Wake up
10.45 a.m.	Pre-nap routine
11.10 a.m.	Active soothing starts
11.30 a.m. to 2.30 p.m.	Nap
Lunch after the nap	
7 p.m.	Dinner followed by the bedtime routine
8.10 p.m.	Active soothing starts
9 p.m.	Asleep for the night

However, if you indeed feel that the fateful time has come to drop the nap, please institute a quiet time (at least one hour in the afternoon in a quiet room, playing with blocks or some other quiet toys, or lying down and cuddling or reading books) just to give the child time to recharge. If the nap is being missed, shift bedtime very early—a little more than 12 hours before the desired morning wakeup time (or 11.5 hours after the morning wake-up that day). Ensure the bedroom is pitch dark and keep the child asleep thereon. For example, if your child's usual morning wake up time is 7 a.m., you should aim for your child to be asleep between 6 and 6.30 p.m. (yes, a very early bedtime). Once she is asleep, please help her to stay asleep by bridging if she tries to wake up thinking it's a nap. It is normal to worry that your child might awake at an ungodly hour in the morning with such an early bedtime, but this is unlikely to happen as children easily clock 12–12.5 hours of sleep at night when they drop the final nap. We can assure you, additionally, that the blissfully early bedtime and having an evening to ourselves as parents are absolutely worth losing our little midday recharge time!

There is likely to be a long period when your child takes a nap on some days and not on other days. Help your child through this. Assess how tired she is. Do the nap if night sleep hasn't been enough or if she is tired for any other reason. If your child is going to school, miss school and do the nap early on such days. For example, if your child has woken up at 5 a.m. one day, don't try to power through the day without a nap and don't do a nap at 1 p.m. after your child returns from school. Follow a 5.5-hours awake window and put your child down for a nap at 10.30 a.m. Assuming your child wakes up by 12.30 p.m., you can still do bedtime 7.5 hours later, at a very reasonable 8 p.m., allowing your child to fall back into a stable no-nap routine the next day. If you feel your child does not need the nap and could power through the day with just a quiet time, help her with that. Avoid a 4 p.m. car drive that could make her nod off. This period requires some management on the part of the parent!

Managing Sleep While Starting School

It can be quite challenging to manage a toddler's sleep if school (including preschool) timings also need to be factored into the mix. Unfortunately, school schedules usually do not align with the biological needs of young children. Keeping this in mind, do consider the question of *when to start school* carefully. We recommend waiting *at least* until the child is on one nap (which happens between 15 and 21 months).

Developmentally, there is much research that states that children do not need school until the age of 4 years or even 6 years (depending on the type of school—and some parents choose not to send their children to school at all by following homeschooling or unschooling). Children do not need school for their intellectual or social development—perhaps ever but certainly not at a young age. Until the age of 3 years, children are socialized beautifully just by seeing their parents interact with others in the normal course of life. They can be taken to playdates, one-off classes, parks. At least until the age of 6 years, they learn best through play and by their imaginations being given free rein.

Parents are often motivated to consider starting school at a young age for a variety of reasons, including the absence of appropriate childcare while parents work, beliefs about the need for socialization or formal learning at a certain age, rigidity in admission processes and stiff competition for seats in the best schools or, sometimes, simply, peer pressure and the rat race. The desirability of starting school late from a developmental perspective is beyond the scope of this book.

However, prioritizing your baby or toddler's *biological* needs over *educational* needs is an important factor when ensuring healthy sleep for your child.

If and when you start school, choose one where the timings suit your child's sleep schedule. The distance of the school from your home can also impact this in a big way. Very often, the timings of the school can delay the single nap of the day. Parents can be tempted to skip the nap to have an early bedtime, or an overtired child may resist the nap and lead the parent to think she is ready to drop the nap. It is not a good idea to skip afternoon naps until children show clear signs that they are ready to drop them—like resisting the nap, having active night wakings, early morning wakings and other signs mentioned earlier in this chapter. Most children do need naps until the age of 4 or 5 years. Dropping the nap should be the child's decision and the child will give clear signs. It should not be the parent's decision, taken to fit a particular schedule, which in this case is school.

For a child to take a nap and also have an early bedtime (and thus get enough sleep at night to wake up fresh the next day for school), the schooltime needs to end early and the nap needs to happen early. As we know, babies are usually ready to take their single naps around 4½–5 hours after morning wakeup at age 2 or 2.5.

For example, Supriya's 2.5-year-old daughter, Aavya, usually woke up at 7.30 a.m. Supriya was very keen to take Aavya to a prestigious preschool 30 minutes away from their house. However, the school's timings were 10.30 a.m. to 1.30 p.m. Supriya was in a dilemma about how to handle this as she knew her daughter would be cranky and tired midway through the class. When she came to Himani for a consultation, Himani explained that this would also lead Aavya to enter an overtired cycle as her nap would start very late, delaying bedtime, leading to disturbed night sleep and also too short a stretch of night sleep, leading to further overtiredness the following day. This was, in truth, going to be a recipe for disaster. Himani gave her two suggestions: one, to find a school where the class ended by noon at the latest and which was nearer home, keeping in mind that, ideally, Aavya should be asleep by noon on days when she awoke at 7.30 a.m. and, even with this preferable school, to try to delay Aavya entering the school by another 6 months when her awake window would expand. In the meanwhile, Supriya could take Aavya to some activity classes in the afternoons after her nap. Supriya took the advice and managed a very smooth transition into schooling over the next 6 months. She enrolled Aavya in activity and music classes 4 days a week, all of which took place after 4 p.m., after a timely and restorative nap. She found a preschool—less famous but equally good—just 10 minutes away from their home. Aavya started there at the age of 3, when her awake window had become 5 hours. The school's timings were 9 a.m. to 12 p.m. Supriya fed Aavya a quick snack in the car on the way back home and had her asleep by 12.45 p.m. Aavya would then wake up by 2.45 p.m. or so and have lunch (see the Chapter 8, 'Your Baby's Sleep: 16 Months to 3 Years', on when to serve lunch) and be ready for bed again by 9.30 p.m., allowing for a good 10-hour stretch of night sleep.

One of the benefits of this routine was that Aavya never had to be woken up. We do not recommend waking a sleeping child under any circumstances—whether in the morning or during the day from the nap. Having to wake a child is a clear indication that the child's sleep needs are not complete and the child will be overtired. So, the child needs to have an early enough bedtime that we are not waking the child up in the morning to be ready for school.

Box 9.1 Our School Has Arrangements for Kids to Nap There. Is That Okay?

Only if they are child-led and responsive and if your child will actually be able to nap there at the right time and for the right length of time. For example, giving children a 45-minute window in which to nap (when a single nap schedule needs a 2–3-hour nap) is not suitable. Many children also need assistance to fall asleep and stay asleep. Many children may also not be able to sleep in a room with light or with other children. It is also important to keep in mind that children under the age of 5 years have to work hard at functioning well in group settings and their internal stress levels can skyrocket if they are left at school for long hours. This can be offset, to an extent, by a nurturing and gentle school environment, but only to an extent.

Is My Child Ready to Sleep in His Own Bed or His Own Room?

Much of our generation grew up sleeping in our parents' beds until the age of 8–9 years and even beyond. The fact is that even most adults prefer to sleep with another human being than alone. As a general recommendation, we would advise waiting until your child asks to sleep in his separate bed or own room. This could happen at 4 years or at 6 years. It could happen at 5 years, then the child could change her mind and stay in the family bed until 7 years. This would be the child-led approach.

Anything parent-led can become easier after 3.5 years and so parents who wish to facilitate a shift to another bed in their room or to another room altogether may find it possible to do so after that age for at least a few hours every night. However, this would not be the child's preferred state in most cases. Even a child who expresses excitement about sleeping separately is unlikely to make it through the night in another bed or another room alone.

If you do wish to shift your toddler to a separate room, the best way to go about it would be to sleep with her in that room for a few weeks or even months. After that, you could stay with her in the room until she falls asleep and then shift back to your room. It would be a good idea to either have a nanny in that room or have a video baby monitor. Your child should always know how to come to you if she so wishes and should always be welcomed in your bed.

Night Terrors and Nightmares

Night terrors and nightmares are two distinct phenomena though both terms are sometimes used to denote bad dreams. Nightmares are the regular bad dreams that afflict all of us. They occur after the age of 2 years at the earliest and take place during REM sleep. Until the age of 6 years, children are not able to distinguish between reality and fantasy. This is why they easily believe in Santa Claus and other fantastical tales. The result is that nightmares are terrifying for them. They seem vivid and real. When children wake up from a nightmare, we recommend you stay calm and offer comfort. If the child is not already in bed with you, take her into bed and cuddle up with her while saying soothing words. If you are breastfeeding, that can be a sure-shot comfort.

If your child is having frequent nightmares, please look into the content your child is watching on television. Something that seems fairly innocuous to us (an old man with a beard for example, or a fox who is preying on a hen) can be terrifying to a toddler. It helps to have conversations about the nightmares they have had, to hear them out without judgement and to acknowledge and validate their feelings with empathy. Something like, 'That must have been very scary for you! You know, I have nightmares too sometimes. I wake up and cuddle your papa/mumma when I do. I know that I am safe in my house and it was just a story in my head, though it seemed so scary. You are also absolutely safe in your bed with us.' Of course, bedsharing does help reduce nightmares. A relaxing bedtime routine can also go a long way to calm a child before night sleep and fill him with love, reassurance and soothing thoughts.

If a child is particularly frightened about nightmares, you can also play some pretend games before bedtime like checking the whole room—behind sofas, under beds—to make sure there are no monsters lurking. You can spray the room with 'anti-nightmare spray' (real or make-believe deodorant!). You can set up a few select stuffed animals who specialize in fighting bad dreams.

Night terrors are quite different and also much less common. They peak between 3 and 8 years of age. They are somewhat like sleep-walking. Your toddler will wake up abruptly from deep sleep, screaming and thrashing. Her eyes will be open but she will not be awake and she will not respond to you. This can last for up to 15 minutes and could happen several times a night. Although this can be very frightening for parents, it is important to stay calm, not intervene and allow the episode to pass. If your child is having night terrors regularly, it is advisable to consult a specialist.

Self-Weaning from Nursing to Sleep

As discussed in the Chapter 8, 'Your Baby's Sleep: 16 Months to 3 Years', the natural age of weaning from breastfeeding is between 3 and 7 years. Babies often wean themselves off nursing to sleep and nursing in general somewhere around this time.

Ramneek Nitesh Gupta, a former admin of GBSI, considered nursing to sleep the bedrock of her sleep management for her twin girls. It was how she managed twin naps, twin bedtimes, twin night wakings, often by herself.

Ramneek shares:

The girls nursed round the clock in the night, meaning every 1–2 hours, till about 24–25 months. After this period, they began to sleep slightly longer stretches—like 2 hours—and so their demand for nursing reduced accordingly. They were continuously latched in the early morning hours till they woke up. This was just our daily story. It is just how they slept during the early morning hours. They have only ever known how to extend sleep with nursing. Regressions, teething and illnesses just added to this. Night weaning them by me was never an option. By tandem nursing them lying down, I could attend to them together at once. How would that work if they both needed comfort and I was not nursing? It was after 30 months that their night feeds came down to barely one–two and they began to prefer snuggling to drinking. Their nursing at night reduced when their sleep became better (and not the other way around) and then stopped once they outgrew a need and decided to seek the comfort they needed another way. Sleep gets better with age as nothing changed in the amount of food they were having before sleep and the amount of physical activity they were getting in the evening in this period. They were also not sleeping through the night most nights. So, nursing to sleep was not connected to sleeping through the night in any way either. At around 38 months, the girls self-weaned off day feeds as well. They mostly fell asleep by themselves with me by their side. Some nights they slept through. Most nights, they came and cuddled me or put their hands or legs under my body, or then asked for me and went right back to sleep hearing me. Indeed, self-weaning was not a myth after all and no bad habits were formed! My girls outgrew nursing to sleep at their own pace.

Sometimes, a little nudge can also be all it takes to move on from nursing to sleep. Neha's son nursed to sleep but was also used to being walked to sleep by his father. Neha tried tentatively to wean at age 2½ years, then 3 years and then at 3½ years by offering walking to sleep by the father instead of nursing. The first two times her son resisted, and Neha immediately reverted to nursing, understanding that he was not ready. It was only at 3.5 years that her son readily accepted moving on from nursing, replaced completely by walking to sleep and patting as the modes of soothing. Soon after, just laying down next to him was enough. The trick is to observe when your child is truly ready. You can choose to do nothing and let nature take its course or you can choose to do the nudge when you feel your child will accept it readily.

10

Sleep for the Modern Parent: How to Handle Family Dynamics and Solo Parenting

All parents struggle with sleep—their own and their baby's—one way or the other. One of the best-kept secrets of a modern parent's life is how to balance it all: restful sleep for the whole family, plenty of exercise, healthy eating, peaceful parenting and a satisfying career. 'Kiss your sleep goodbye!' or 'Sleep now as much as you can because when the baby comes, you won't get any!' are comments that come at you fast and furious as a to-be-parent. Despite all the half-truthful warnings, nothing prepares you for what happens when the baby comes along.

An infant likes to sleep most of the day and as she grows, her sleep needs change. She requires more careful monitoring to watch for early sleep cues, like rubbing of eyes and ears, eyes glazing over, looking distracted or hungry, and needs a quiet, dark environment to sleep, as adults do too. But very often, parents misread the signs. No one tells them that to help your baby sleep, you need to make certain modifications to your home, to your routine and listen to your baby.

Our GBSI Survey reveals that over 40 per cent of parents did not know anything about baby sleep before they joined GBSI. Most parents believe that babies sleep whenever they want. Babies are indeed born with an inbuilt ability to fall asleep, but modern life creates many hurdles for them. In ancient times, a natural setting of the forest, with few things to keep early humans frantically busy, allowed for the body to slow down at will at the first sign of sleep.

In our busy modern lives, though, we are always trying to do more than is humanly possible. We send our bodies signals that keep it awake, instead of slowing down when it's time to sleep or when we feel tired. We spend our days in a stress-induced haze, barely clocking 6–7 hours of sleep at night. One of the major factors that causes ups and downs in the world of baby sleep is, indeed, tied to the many relentless demands of modern life.

You know how complicated our days tend to get: doorbells ringing early morning to signal the arrival of house help or groceries, getting breakfast on the table in time to make it for the morning meeting, a cranky baby who is looking ready for a nap for whom you are trying to quickly rustle up an age-appropriate meal, putting the baby down for a nap only to have him up in 20 minutes, meal-planning and prepping for the rest of the day, more naps, park and playtime, finishing up more chores, answering emails, calls, attending meetings and, if that isn't enough, scheduling fun activities for the baby (and you!). By the end of the day, you are trying the best you can to stay calm and cheerful through dinner to make it to bedtime, which your child seems to resist as well. A quick tip here: Your child and you are inexplicably connected. Our lives as adults are so deeply tied to theirs as children that very often sleep resistance or sleep concerns cannot be explained in terms of age-appropriate sleep and routines—it is so much about how the day has gone, the time you have spent with your child and your overall style of parenting. Think of it like a complex, challenging puzzle for which you need all the pieces to come together at the end of the day. One of the pieces of the puzzle is routines.

If you're wondering where's the time to *think* about sleep, much less bother about routines, we absolutely get your worries.

Our busy, packed, modern lives make it difficult to dedicate the time and energy it takes to help a baby get age-appropriate rest, especially with small family structures and fewer hands to help. But take it from us: investing time in it at this early stage makes life easier as children grow. While many parents believe spending time and effort on figuring out baby sleep is not practical and too all-consuming, the opposite is true—the more effort you make to understand the nuances of biological sleep needs in the first 2 years, the less complicated your life will be going forward. A modern-day parent's secret weapon is routines, without which it's usually chaos. Nobody wants their children to be perpetually sleep-deprived, but over 80 per cent of Indian children are, and this is preventable.

As parents in a wildly changing world, we have many rivers to cross: rising above the challenges of a nuclear family, with both parents working, how to manage baby sleep as a solo parent, how to figure out a reasonable routine living abroad with no family or paid help, how to get the baby to sleep well while travelling, how to say yes to dinner invitations that clash with bedtime and, one of the most befuddling of all, how to get the father of the child, the co-parent, onboard the baby sleep wagon.

Here's the good news: you *can* have it all if you make some crucial modifications.

To get there, let's take you through the nitty-gritty of how life can look once you add your baby's sleep routine to your daily calendar.

Nuclear Family Conundrum

With just two adults to manage children, work and housekeeping, lack of sleep can make life a lot more difficult. But careful planning can go a long way. Let's start at the beginning. Consider the fact that most women are given maternity leave of four to six months if they are working outside the home. This leave can be used fruitfully to get your baby into an age-appropriate routine, while offering unconditional, unhindered attachment that offers the baby deep safety and security to be able to instinctually stay asleep. Using the SHARED method (as explained in Chapter 3, 'How to Get Your Baby to Sleep: The SHARED Method', watch for early sleep cues, hold for naps and lie down with your baby so she feels secure enough to continue sleeping.

In our survey, over 50 per cent of mothers reported that their biggest sleep issue is that their baby naps very little during the day and goes to bed very late at night and resists sleep at all times. This can be particularly trying for a nuclear family because a cranky, overtired baby who sleeps very little is a recipe for disaster—there is no alternate caregiver to offer respite unless you have paid help who is good with the baby.

Why do most infants find it difficult to nap and have a restful night sleep? The reason is rather simple and goes back to our basic instincts. It's because they are not kept close enough to a caregiver, especially the mother, to sleep. Babies need lots and lots of secure attachment, skin to skin contact and literally need to be joined at the hip for at least the first few months to one or two primary caregivers.

When provided with a secure attachment, watch as your baby will fall into a routine on her own because you spent the first few months both physically and mentally completely connected, treating her like an extension of yourself. This gives the baby deep confidence to be at peace with her surroundings and satiates her survival instincts. It makes her feel safe enough to sleep.

In her revolutionary book *The Continuum Concept*, author Jean Liedloff writes: 'It's perfectly clear that the millions of babies, who are crying at this very moment, want unanimously to be next to a live body. Do you really think they're all wrong? Theirs is the voice of nature. This is the clear, pure voice of nature, without intellectual interference.' Listening to your child's leads, every cry, every need is what ensures that as the baby grows, he becomes more cooperative and understanding and far better adjusted than a baby who hasn't got enough sleep and is cranky and unable to regulate his emotions.

From a practical point of view, charting out a routine that is worked around the baby's nap and bedtime would allow a nuclear family to thrive and grow with the baby. So, for example, both parents could work around their schedules in a way that doesn't clash with the baby's sleep routine. Hiring the best help you can afford (including a reliable, gentle nanny) is a personal choice depending on one's financial situation and other factors. But it does pay off to have a helper around if you look at it as an investment to run a home smoothly without stressing out the mother and to allow for downtime.

When Neha gave birth to her son in 2014, she had about 4 months' maternity leave. She and her husband did not have family members living close by who could pitch in with regular childcare. They hired a housekeeper and a cook who took care of their needs during the day while Neha and her husband took care of the baby. Essentially, they focused on staying close to the baby all the time. Neha held him for naps on her lap, propped up with a nursing pillow, books close at hand. She wore him in an ergonomic baby carrier when he was awake and went about her chores, grocery shopping and walks in the park. When her husband was home during the day on holidays, their son would nap on his chest. On other days, Neha handed him over to her husband every evening when he came home from work. He spent time with their son, fed him a bottle of milk and walked him to sleep after that. When their son stirred at night, Neha fed him back to sleep. When their son crossed the 4-month mark and entered his first regression that came with frequent wakings and troubled nights, Neha's husband walked the baby back to sleep when he didn't want to nurse. By the time he was 5 months old, their son was doing longer naps and that allowed Neha to start working from home when he napped peacefully next to her and played with the helper when awake. He was sleeping 10–12 hours at night (waking briefly for feeds and comforting) and was a happy, active baby who took three to four naps during the day. Their days were predictable and moved like clockwork. This happened because they had made their child's sleep a priority and figured out a way to make the rest of the to-dos align with it. This meant that their routine changed slightly to keep up with their child's changing sleep needs as he grew. They planned their outings when he was awake. Now that their son is older and an independent sleeper who still loves his sleep and clocks in the recommended hours at night, it's easy to see how the years they invested in inculcating healthy sleep habits played a massive role in shaping his most important developmental years.

In short, figure out an age-appropriate sleep routine (follow our suggested schedules in Chapter 4, 'What Baby Sleep Looks Like: The Sleep Pyramid') for your child and plan your day around it. You will thank us later.

Returning to Work

Responding to your child's sleep needs is relatively easy when one or both parents is home on maternity or paternity break. That break is meant to help you connect with your baby and take tiny steps into parenthood. But much of that time becomes terribly stressful for parents today because they worry about how their kids will adjust once they are no longer around to offer special attention and care as they return to work. This is a very valid concern. Alternate caregivers may or may not be able to offer the same kind of support, especially when it comes to sleep. Mothers, especially, feel jittery about going back to an office and being cut off from their baby after just a few months of full-time parenting. It's definitely very hard to detach yourself when the first few months your life revolved around your little one. Mothers often wonder how their nursing babies will be able to sleep without breastfeeding to sleep, without their touch and undivided attention. However, we are here to assure you that it is perfectly possible to go back to work AND have your baby do well sleep-wise, without having to wean from the breast. What you need is meticulous planning and a solid support system. Some of the common concerns we come across are:

- If I nurse my baby to sleep throughout my maternity break, how will the baby adjust when I go back to office? Should I stop nursing to sleep?

- If I create quiet and dark rooms for the baby to sleep in when I am home and hold the baby for naps, how will my baby learn to sleep in different sleep environments with different caregivers?
- How will my baby adjust to bottle-feeding if I feed on demand directly from the breast to aid sleep?

The golden rule of parenting is to go with the flow. Nothing ever remains the same in babyland, so don't worry too much if your baby is used to a certain way of sleeping right now. Babies live in phases. What works one month may not work the next. So, if you have to return to work in a few months, enjoy your time with the baby now and continue doing what works, whether that is nursing/rocking/walking to sleep, even as you prepare for a gentle transition to other caregivers. Of course, it is important to choose a reliable and sensitive caregiver who will understand and respect your child's needs in your absence. You will need to train the new caregiver in your child's age-appropriate sleep routine and help him/her figure out the best mode of soothing that works for your baby. But the good news is that babies do adjust to new situations well when given the chance, enough time and offered a good enough replacement for you. Expect your baby to take two to four weeks at the minimum to adjust. Think of it like a new job or a new house—wouldn't you need enough time to settle in? Babies need time to make sense of new arrangements too. Try to ensure that the alternate caregiver is in the baby's orbit one to two months before you plan to go back to work so there is enough time for the child to learn to trust the new caregiver. Have the baby play with the new caregiver in your presence. It will be much easier for a new caregiver to help the baby sleep if the child has grown accustomed to his/her presence and place in the house. Do not expect a baby to suddenly take to a new nanny or new caregiver at a daycare within a day or two. Let's remember that a baby's basic instincts are very strong and they absolutely have no reason to trust a near stranger; so, they will feel stressed and even traumatized when expected to feel secure with a new person taking care of them. A gentle and slow transition goes a long way in ensuring that your own journey back to work is smooth and drama-free and you are able to return to a happy, well-rested child every evening.

Let's consider the example of Divya Chandrahas Mehta, a finance professional in Mumbai, who returned to her job when her child was 7 months old.

> We hired a nanny when he was about 5.5 months old. So, roughly, I had about 1.5 months to get him used to pumped milk (using a bottle) and for the nanny to put him to bed. Initially, it was met with a lot of resistance. But, he would take a bottle if I stepped out briefly. The nanny also figured out that walking and singing was what he was comfortable with to go off to sleep. I had briefed her about awake windows, holding for naps. And while she was initially hesitant to hold for naps, eventually, she realized, that was the only way he would sleep longer. I would come home during lunch hours to feed. I also pumped at work for around 7 months and used to drop off the milk pouches during lunch hours. I continued to nurse him to sleep whenever I was around at home, and at night.

Here is another scenario, where a grandparent was left in charge of the baby, with a helper to assist in the heavy lifting, which caring for a child can definitely be! Himani Dhaundiyal devised a step-by-step transition to help her son adjust to his grandmother and also a helper. 'For naps, I started with nursing him to sleep, and then having the caregiver hold him for naps.

Then I gradually moved to nursing my baby a bit before naptime and then handing him over to the caregiver to rock to sleep. Simultaneously, I also had the baby get used to taking milk from the bottle from the caregiver. Then, I started stepping out of the house during naptime.' Her baby soon started associating rocking/walking/swaying to sleep with the caregiver, and nursing to sleep with her. She found it was very important for the baby to be comfortable and familiar with the caregiver. 'I started around 5–6 weeks before joining work, and gradually moved from one stage to another. It takes a few weeks for sure, and sleep does take a bit of a hit initially. But babies adjust very well if we do it gradually and gently, and give them time to adjust,' she adds.

Box 10.1 Making It Work with a Nanny: Himani's Story

Himani and Akash chose not to hire a full-time nanny as they found that they preferred to handle the baby themselves. When their first daughter, Devika, was born, they had a lady, Mamta (name changed), who had worked in their home for 4 years already in a housekeeper-like role. Himani and Akash lived in a nuclear family set-up and Mamta was of immense support to the parents as they nursed the baby, held the baby, bathed the baby and did all the primary caregiving. Mamta could bring Himani her food and water, manage the baby's room and clothing and entertain the baby for a few minutes at a time if Himani needed to use the bathroom or eat a meal and Akash was at work. Over time, Himani and Akash found that the housekeeper had a wonderful knack and gentle touch with the baby. She could easily rock the baby to sleep and keep her asleep by holding her. Himani worked in her own business at that time and started visiting the office for a few hours every day after Devika turned 6 months old. She converted a cabin next to hers into a makeshift nursery with a little playpen, toy box, playmat, blackout blinds and comfortable seating. She took Devika with her, along with Mamta. Himani could work in her cabin while Devika played with Mamta. Himani would nurse the baby and then Mamta would hold her for her nap. When their second daughter, Yamini, was born, Mamta's support proved invaluable, especially when Akash was not at home, as she could hold the newborn for naps while Himani spent time with the toddler. Alternatively, Mamta could play with the toddler while Himani nursed and held the newborn. The ratio of three adults to two babies proved very helpful! At the same time, Mamta's housekeeping responsibilities continued and she was not a full-time nanny. Himani and Akash continued to do the bulk of caregiving, from bathing to feeding to holding to playing to managing bedtime and all nighttime parenting, with Mamta pitching in as and when required. This system worked well for Himani and Akash as it allowed them to practise the kind of hands-on parenting that came naturally to them while also balancing work and caring for siblings with a short age difference.

The Joint Family Dilemma

Living in a joint family can be a huge support—and also challenging. It's never easy to have all family members on board with your preferred style of parenting. Frequent conflicts over what works best for the baby are common, so if you've had them too, you are not alone. Many parents come to us for support when their efforts to follow a routine do not appeal to grandparents or other caregivers. This can be a source of frequent friction. There are bound to be generational differences in how to bring up the baby. Our parents and grandparents parented in a different time when 'sleep science' was an alien concept and they had many other worries that kept them occupied. Children slept when they fell asleep out of exhaustion. And everyone just got on with it. They didn't know any better. They had uniquely different pressures. In many cases, they lived in large families where one child had several caregivers. It was quite the norm to put babies into cradles or swings, often made out of saris, hung from the ceiling. It also wasn't uncommon to use sleep-inducing medicines or herbal remedies for babies. None of these methods is considered safe any longer. Today's joint family looks distinctly different. Families are smaller, tighter units today, and we look more towards screens for entertainment and comfort than ever before. The advent of screens plays havoc with a child's sleep.

A modern parent has many battles to fight. Now, with considerable research and evidence on age-appropriate sleep at our disposal, it wouldn't be wise to ignore the fact that sleep too needs your urgent attention. So how can you wade through the family clashes over sleep?

Sample one query we received: 'How do you guys manage baby sleep in a joint family setup? My in-laws pounce on the baby the moment she opens her eyes, irrespective of whether she has woken up or (her sleep) needs bridging. They keep playing with the baby until my baby gets irritated, and when the time comes to put her to sleep, my mother-in-law hands her back to me saying she seems hungry. I dread when someone enters the room and I know that the time to bridge is near. Adding to the agony are the innumerable visitors popping up at nap timings and entering the room making loud noises!'

Sounds familiar? It's a situation that many parents face, especially when their babies are very young. Tradition dictates that the needs of elders in the family must come first, even if it makes children cranky, overtired and miss their naps. But many parents, with our guidance, managed to convince their family members that following an age-appropriate sleep routine, keeping screens off or volume low as much as possible during sleep time and catching early sleep cues is the right way to go. One of the tricks that helped was to take them along for the ride, by sharing articles and research with them (or this book!) that speak of the advantages of healthy sleep for babies. If that doesn't work—and often elders would look dismissively at what they believe is new-age nonsense—you may need to stand up for your baby, and agree to disagree in a peaceful way. After all, this is your time to do things the way you believe is best for your baby. Let them know you respect their opinion and approach and it may have worked well in their time. If you see a sliver of interest from their end, add them to GBSI on Facebook. We are happy to have grandparents on board! Another way to show them that following routines and gentle baby sleep methods work is to tell them to leave it to you for a month, even as an experiment. As your child's sleep improves, they are bound to be taken in. It may take time, but in the end, it will be worth it. After all, let's remember the entire family wants the best for the child, even if the way to get there is somewhat unconventional.

Flying Solo: Making It Work as a Single Parent

A wise person once said that solo parenting is twice the work, twice the stress and twice the tears, but it's also twice the hugs, twice the love and twice the pride. Sneha Jain Ashok, a young single parent to a 27-month-old feisty toddler, knows exactly what that means. She has been raising her daughter with the help of her parents after she separated from her husband. She joined GBSI when her baby was around 10 months old. What helped her get her daughter's routine in place was taking baby steps towards understanding the nuances of sleep, which kept her from becoming overwhelmed during the difficult phases.

This is what she says about the process of getting there:

> I didn't realize, before learning about it from the group, that we can be tuned in to our baby's sleep cues and pay attention to how long she is awake. I inculcated a good winding down pre-nap routine, like giving a massage and a shower, changing her clothes and nursing her to sleep. I also made a lot of changes in the room after learning that babies need a dark and calm environment to sleep. I got blackout curtains and white noise. I tried the 2–3–4 sleep pattern which is meant for children on two naps, and it worked like a charm! I would stay next to my daughter during her naps and bridged her sleep whenever she stirred. Meanwhile, my mother took care of the home and made sure my daughter's sleep routine wasn't affected in any way. My father has also been very supportive—he always asked me about my daughter's nap timings and refrained from playing with her when it might be time for the nap. My parents also helped me a lot especially during regressions, early morning wakings and night wakings, taking over whenever I needed to sleep.

Solo parenting can be very rewarding and empowering: you call the shots on your baby's routine and there is less interference from people around—most of the time at least! But, of course, it can be overwhelming and exhausting dealing with sleep deprivation and the emotional rollercoaster that early parenting can be.

What will make your life as a single parent easier, as illustrated by Sneha's case, is not being harsh on yourself or trying to do everything on your own. As you focus on developing an age-appropriate routine once your child crosses the 2–3-month mark, do not feel shy to enlist whatever support you can find—from grandparents, other parents or paid support. If you need to go into an office, finding a good daycare or a nanny who understands your needs as a parent will ensure less stress for you. If you work from home, then having someone take care of the home chores and childcare while you oversee the routine can go a long way. As a single parent, you need to invest in taking care of your own needs as much as your baby's.

Box 10.2 Can Sleeping with Your Baby Kill Your Marriage?

The renowned Spanish paediatrician and bestselling parenting author Carlos González dedicated a small but precious section in his wonderfully insightful book *Kiss Me!: How to Raise Your Children with Love* to this befuddling question that troubles many parents, though far more so in the West. In the section 'Children, beds and sex', he writes:

> They say that a baby in the bedroom interferes with a couple's sex life. But that isn't true. When babies sleep they sleep so very deeply; and when the baby sleeps in his parents' bed it is possible, once he is asleep, to take him out and put him in his

cot for a while. Of course, he may wake up suddenly, but that can also happen if he sleeps in a separate room, and if no one goes running to him, in two minutes he will be screaming his head off. Besides, the day is long and the house has many rooms. If you can't find a way of having sexual relations, don't blame it on your child.

Putting a child in a separate room, claim many sleep trainers, can save your relationship after having a baby. This argument is riddled with holes. The suggestion that babies should be expected to sleep alone, something that goes completely against their instinct, so that two adults can enjoy intimacy sounds not only patently absurd but also ridiculously silly. The truth is that parenthood can certainly threaten an already troubled marriage. If things were tough before you had a baby, it's unlikely to get better after having a baby, simply because parenting can be a deeply demanding, immensely exhausting and seemingly endless phase that can test the patience of even the most saintly. So naturally, a weak relationship riddled with problems is going to be further challenged. However, a strong, solid marriage based on equal or near-equal participation of both parents in caring for their child, built on mutual respect and deep love is likely to become even better when you connect over nurturing a little one. You don't need us to tell you that having an active sex life and open communication has little to do with having complete control over one room or bed in the house. If your relationship feels like it needs saving, if there is a lack of connection, especially after having a child, sending your baby to another room isn't going to solve it. You could consider marriage counselling and taking out time to talk (respectful discussions can certainly happen while your baby is around too!). Further, having a well-rested, well-respected baby feeds into a good marriage, leads to fewer clashes and certainly does not take away from it. As celebrity actor Mayim Bialik of *The Big Bang Theory* fame, a longtime supporter of bedsharing, once said: 'Worried about your fantastic sex life taking a hit? Find other places to have sex besides your bed.' Get creative! And you'll have plenty to bond over.

11

Sleep on the Go: Travelling, Moving Abroad and Having a Social Life

As a modern parent, life can often be unpredictable. There are fewer hands and increasing responsibilities. Often, there is the danger of your childcare support system falling apart just when you need it the most. With demanding home chores and career challenges, your days with a child can feel chaotic. Add stepping out of your comfort zone to the mix and it's easy to feel overwhelmed. This chapter is designed to help you dial back on your anxiety and make it easier for you to understand how sleep works when you are outside your home, the space most familiar to you and your baby.

Sleeping on an Airplane

Have you ever worried that travelling with a baby could turn out to be a nightmare? Have you had a difficult experience doing it before? It doesn't have to be this way. We all need breaks from our hectic lives and having a baby doesn't mean you shouldn't pack your bags and put your travelling shoes on. And just because you're travelling doesn't mean your baby's sleep will go for a toss.

So how do you ensure that a holiday is indeed a holiday, without meltdowns because of lack of sleep? The trick is to remember that even if you are on vacation, your child still definitely needs his routine.

Sure, the sound of routines while on holiday can seem oppressive and annoying. But routines are the bedrock of every community across the world and for every age group. Routines bind our days together, stitching them into a whole and helping us make sense of an otherwise chaotic world. What makes routines special is that they are predictable, reliable, offering security and safety while inducing confidence, cooperation and connection. If you think about it, you would have almost always had a routine since you were a baby, through your teens and adulthood, consciously or, more often, unconsciously. This is because the human body is designed and equipped to function most successfully when it is aligned with the rising and setting of the sun. Research has widely proven that those who follow regular routines have better sleep cycles and emotional regulation.

When given the right environment, we function on a routine in autopilot, leaving our brain free to work through daily conundrums and creative challenges without becoming overburdened. You will notice you feel hungry, sleepy and in the need of a bathroom visit around the same time every day. When you miss a meal or sleep later than usual, you tend to feel out of sync and unable to focus and move around with the usual ease.

It's pretty much the same with children. In fact, children need routines even more than adults because they are more vulnerable to the negative effects of sleep deprivation and lack the ability to regulate themselves as their stress levels rise, which happens as a consequence of missed naps and delayed bedtime.

Holidays are no different. Children (and adults) need a routine on holiday too, with some flexibility. When children are out of their comfort zone and stimulated by a new environment as they tend to be while on holiday, the routine becomes their safe place. The closer you stick to the child's usual routine while on holiday, the smoother your trip is likely to be. It's true that children adapt to different places well, but not when they are sleep-deprived and cranky. Your child is going to love splashing about in the pool, running around at the beach and taking in the many wondrous sights when out if she has had her nap(s) for the day. Additionally, you don't want to deviate from the routine too much while travelling because then when you are back home it is going to be doubly hard to adjust to the usual sleep timings. Here are some tips for how you can make it happen:

1. **CARRY:** Pack an ergonomic baby carrier that the baby can nap in when you are on the move. Prams are useful too, but babies usually nap better when they feel close to the caregiver in a carrier, especially when you are in motion or in noisy places such as at an airport.

2. **PLAN:** Design your travel itinerary in a way that allows your baby to sleep on the move. If driving, help the baby nap in the car at his usual time. Book flights at a time that would allow him to nap during the journey. Try and do day flights rather than night journeys when travelling within the country. When doing long flights to international destinations, try and take a night flight so that your child can do a nice long stretch of sleep at his usual time to sleep. Nurse/hold baby for naps at the regular bedtime, or close to

it. Younger babies may adjust well in a bassinet too, so be sure to book one in advance.

3. **BOOK:** When booking a hotel room, get a king-size bed. Try and get back to the room at naptime. A couple of naps on the move are fine while babywearing or in a pram so that the child can fall asleep while you walk. But try and be back to the hotel by the time bedtime rolls around. We have taken plenty of memorable holidays, right from when our babies were a few months old, without disturbing their routine. Once the babies were sound asleep in bed, we had a little private celebration of our own - adults only! And the kids were raring to go the next day after a great night's sleep. So were we.

Box 11.1 Himani's Travel Tip

When Himani and Akash travelled after becoming parents, they always ensured that they had a living arrangement where they could step out somewhere after the baby was asleep. Their babies had early bedtimes and slept in a pitch dark and quiet room. The parents needed to step out of the bedroom after 8 p.m. to eat dinner and have some leisure time. If they were staying with family or friends, this was not a problem. They also planned trips with grandparents so that the parents could go to the grandparents' room after bedtime. If travelling by themselves, they always ensured they booked a suite, even if that meant choosing a lower category hotel or an apartment or reworking their annual holiday budget to include one less trip! It was simply not an option for them to live in a single room any more.

Moving Abroad

Living under circumstances that are culturally and geographically removed from your own can seem daunting and confusing, especially as a new parent. Instinctively, you could be drawn to parenting philosophies you would have seen around you growing up in India, but the parenting culture and social pressures of the country of your new residence can play a significant role in how you approach the challenges of baby sleep too.

On GBSI, we try to address the concerns of parents not just in India but also those who log in from across the world to post their urgent queries. We try to bring them in touch with the very basic instincts and parental impulses that remain the same no matter where you live or which culture you identify with.

However, living abroad does come with its unique challenges. You often have little or no paid help. Parents are sometimes confused about how to manage holding their child for naps or bridging sleep cycles when they have many chores to finish. They are stressed about having to cook or turn up at work the day after frequent night wakings when they have very little family support to give them a breather during difficult periods such as sleep regressions, growth spurts and developmental milestones. Often, these concerns overlap with the challenges that parents face anywhere, but the isolation of being away from the hustle and bustle of India, with its uniquely resourceful system, can be particularly challenging.

There is a dangerous myth though that if you live abroad with no help, you must sleep-train your child. Many parents have been misled into believing that for their sanity and in the best interest of their children's safety, they must leave the child to cry to sleep on a separate sleeping surface.

This is a claim that holds no weight. While the medical systems in many Western countries do recommend that you keep a separate room ready and fitted with a crib before the baby is brought home, there is no reason to not bedshare while following all safety rules and attend to your child even if there is a nursery in the house. The nursery, after all, can be a lovely space to play during the day and offer the child a bright, cheerful spot to call her own. But as a parent, it is your prerogative where your child sleeps and it is up to you to make that decision, not your doctor or your child's paediatrician. So, it is perfectly healthy to bedshare even if you live abroad (where culturally it may be more common to have babies sleeping in a crib) while keeping in mind all safe sleeping practices. (See Chapter 12, 'The Sleep Training Trap and the Myth of Self-Soothing'.)

The formula to cracking the gentle baby sleep code while living without help is to adopt the two P's: Planning and Preparation.

Mallika Ramaswamy, who lives in Sydney, Australia, and has been part of the admin team on GBSI, is an attached and gentle parent to two kids, 4½ and 2 years old, and vouches for the fact that it is possible to make it work. Here's her toolkit for harried parents:

It is really difficult to have to juggle work and kids. But with a few tricks, a lot of support and determination, it is completely doable. First, I think it is really important to have everyone around you on the same page on your baby's sleep, especially if one of your family (like mother/mother-in-law) is going to look after your baby in your absence. So, do tackle that first. If your baby's sleep is your priority, everything else takes a backseat. I always try and revolve everything around my children's naps. My husband manages a lot of housework, especially over the weekends, so we share the load. On my days off work, I try to make work lunches, meal prep a little, finish up laundry and cleaning, so I am available to the kids the rest of the time. Both my children have needed a caregivers' physical presence to nap, so my husband and I make sure that at least one of us is with them. With both my babies, I started work only after they were 1–1.5 years old, so they had very predictable routines, to begin with. Also, my husband and mother/mother-in-law were their alternate caregivers and could get them to sleep from a very young age. My husband was always a very hands-on father and took responsibility for the babies' sleep from Day 1 of their birth. He would get them to sleep for their weekend naps, and some weekday nights as well. When both my kids were about 6 months old, my mother-in-law also started getting them to sleep. This was very helpful when I started work. Initially, I would leave them with her to bridge the nap only, and slowly they got comfortable enough to do the entire nap with her. Finally, from about a month to when I had to join work, they did about six to eight hours with her. That helped her get comfortable with them and also gave me the confidence to get back to work without worrying much about them, knowing that they would sleep well.

Thousands of miles away in Canada, Himani Dhaundiyal, another admin member of GBSI, has similar priorities. She moved from Delhi to Ottawa when her son Ahaan was 18 months old.

It was a huge change from having family and paid help around almost all the time to being completely on our own. The key for us was to really set our priorities. Sleep had to be at the top for this to work. Everything else came later. It took some planning, dividing of tasks and trying to stick to the plan as much as possible. For example, making a meal plan and prepping/cooking most of it over the weekend—that was me. Meal plans were simplified too: they had to be nutritionally balanced, but not elaborate. After that, I didn't have to spend more than 20–30 minutes putting together meals during weekdays. Lunch was always leftovers from dinner. Cleaning the entire house over the weekend was done by my husband, Deepak. Minimizing our clutter, no fancy stuff at the house helped. There were fewer things to clean. Deepak took care of breakfast before leaving for work and took over Ahaan after he got back in the evening. Tasks like doing the dishes and cleaning the kitchen were done after Ahaan went to bed. I could do simple tasks like folding laundry, putting together a salad while sitting next to Ahaan and talking to him.

Since by that time I could leave Ahaan for the first 90 minutes of his nap, I would take that time to catch up on any chores like doing the laundry, any spot cleaning, or just have a cup of coffee in peace. The second half of his nap, I would either nap after bridging his nap or just lie down next to him or catch up with reading or Netflix. Those 60–90 mins of relaxing in the middle of the day were crucial. What also helped me cope was an outing by myself or with a friend at least once a month, sometimes twice on a weekend, where I did not have to take care of naptime as well. There were, of course, days when the best-laid plans went awry, the dishes piled up, the house looked like it had been hit by a hurricane and it was hard to ignore the mess, but we just gave each other extra reminders of what was more important at the end of the day, and that helped.

Another important consideration for parents moving abroad is tackling bedtime in summers. If you move to a country closer to the poles, you will encounter longer days, when even 9 p.m. will seem like daytime. This can make the process of getting the child ready for bedtime challenging. What can help is finding the right kind of curtains for your room. We faced this during our first summer in Canada and quickly realized that just making the bedroom pitch dark won't work because your child can see that it's very bright outside when you tell him it's bedtime. So, we invested in thick dark curtains for all rooms, just for summers. Drawing those curtains right before dinner signalled that it's getting dark and we're approaching bedtime. Also the bedtime routine took slightly longer for us in summers, so we had to start it a bit earlier.

Toddlers may find the longer summer days more stimulating than babies, so it's good to factor that in and build the routine and sleep environment wherever you are moving to accordingly.

Box 11.2 Managing Jetlag

Jetlag refers to disturbed sleep that you experience once you travel quickly across time zones. Your body clock still functions as per the time zone you travelled from and takes a few days before you get acclimatized to the new time zone. Jetlag affects babies even more than it affects adults and may take 7–10 days before the effects wear out.

Nidhi Doshi, a parent to a 5-year-old child who is based in Canada, managed her son's sleep routine through long-distance travel between India and the US, beating jet lag and moving home across countries. How did she do it? Hear it from her.

What to expect:

1. Frequent night wakings and active wakings that might last a few hours.
2. Long naps at odd times of the day.
3. Sudden drop or increase in appetite.
4. Baby will be clingier than usual.

Why does this happen?

This is all a part of the settling process and will usually self-correct within a few days with a good routine as the baby gets acquainted with the new environment. During this time, the baby might be cranky or seek lots of comfort from the parent.

How can we help them?

1. For the first few days, try to follow a schedule similar to the one you did before moving. The primary target for the first few days should be to help the baby get sufficient rest to overcome the exhaustion from a long flight.
2. Make sure the baby isn't overtired by watching out for early sleep cues and following an age-appropriate waketime and nap schedule. Don't look at the time on the clock, but follow the wake windows that suit the age of the child till the timings self-correct in about a week or 10 days.

3. Start following a bedtime routine again to indicate night even if the baby is active and not exactly sleepy. Schedules are bound to go haywire while suffering from jet lag, so, try to move back into rhythm at a pace that the baby and you are comfortable with.

4. Help babies correct their circadian rhythm by allowing lots of light and sound during the day (though not during naps) and by keeping the room dark and quiet at night.

5. Give your little one lots and lots of cuddles, hold them and be by their side as the parent is the only comfort that they have in an unknown environment. Clinginess is very common during such a time. Try getting sufficient rest when the baby rests to help you recover from jet lag as well. Being well-rested will help you deal with night wakings. As always, both parents being involved in sorting sleep out and sharing the burden of jetlag is best. Enlisting help from your family if they are around can ease this bumpy period too.

Having a Social Life

The invitation arrived in Neha's inbox just as her son turned 4 months old. 'It's our 10th wedding anniversary! You must come (with the baby of course!).' Neha looked around frantically for the time of the party. 'Cocktails and dinner start at 9 p.m.', it said. In their post-baby life, 9 p.m. was like midnight—way too late for any kind of socializing. There was no doubt in Neha's mind that this party wasn't going to be feasible for them. It was past her son's bedtime and it would be a huge disruption for him to be taken to a noisy dinner. A few weeks later, however, they received another invitation for a cosy gathering at a former coworker's home across town. 'Can we make it an early evening?' Neha asked. 'Of course,' she said, and sportingly made arrangements for an early dinner and readied a room so Neha's son could take a nap in between the conversations. And just like that, they had a great time together with the least disruption for the baby's sleep and Neha was back home just as his bedtime rolled around. Everyone slept well that night.

It all ties into one of our most important baby sleep recommendations: let your outings never clash (unless it is an emergency of some kind) with your child's sleep routine. Stepping out with your baby when it's time for him to sleep is quite like stepping into quicksand: you won't come out of it in one piece! It leads to crankiness, overtiredness and a disturbed routine which is likely to cause more night wakings than usual with a loss of emotional regulation—for both you and your baby.

Naturally, most parents find that their social life is considerably altered after a baby lands in the mix. It needn't be cause for alarm or distress, however. It can be an opportunity to explore the novelty of a different kind of social life that you can map based on your child's routine at that time and your bandwidth. It's fun all the same—just a different kind of fun!

Himani, for example, finds her social interactions have shifted to lunches and teas on the weekend after having her two children. 'We do drinks and/or dinner at my own house. It takes a little coming to terms with but, honestly, it's worth it to not mess with the baby's schedule! Things get a little easier around the 18–20-month mark, and the occasional late night doesn't affect them too much, I believe. Until then, I would just master the art of declining invitations,' she says.

We realize there is no one-size-fits-all approach, of course. Some families are more social than others and have varying degrees of obligations and priorities. Depending on your situation and family dynamic, here are some tips you could use to tweak your social life which allow you to let down your hair while also keeping the baby's sleep routine front and centre:

1. **Choose well.** In the first few years, accept social invitations that are truly important to you and offer you some leeway in terms of time and day.

2. **Become the host.** As Himani said, move the party to your house. Put the baby to bed, press play on the white noise, keep the baby monitor next to you and hang out with your friends and family.

3. **Pivot.** Accept that your social life will change after having a baby, and that's a good thing. It means everyone is growing up, not just the baby! Request friends and family to be flexible and accommodate celebrations at a time in the day that are baby-friendly. And while your outings may seem severely limited in the first year or so, once the baby moves to a one nap routine (at around 15–18 months), it gets a lot easier to plan visits.

4. **Take turns.** If there are invitations you do not want to decline that clash with your baby's sleep routine, take turns to go. You attend one while your spouse goes to the next one, or one that is more important to either one of you.

5. **Get your me-time.** Once your baby's routine has settled down, go out with your friends while your partner does bedtime and bridges sleep cycles. For this to happen successfully, involve your partner in baby sleep from Day 1.

6. **Create your 'outing' at home**. If it's hard to go out or you just feel too exhausted to leave home, staying in can be just as fun. Snuggle up with the latest Netflix movie or your favourite book, a tub of popcorn and your beverage of choice once your baby is down for the night. Now that the COVID-19 pandemic has made virtual parties legitimate social events—go right ahead and organize your own Zoom gatherings.

7. **It's all a phase.** Hitting pause on late-night socializing pays off in the end, we promise you. Sticking around to help your baby sleep at night rather than taking her out with you when it's her bedtime results in a well-rested child who grows to love her sleep because she is in touch with her internal cues and feels safe and cared for. As she grows, you will be able to socialize more without compromising on her sleep.

8. **Find your tribe.** In the time of social media, it's easy to find a tribe of your kind of parents who are happy to create fun social experiences that are planned to suit baby routines. Look around and reach out to them! Take turns to plan gatherings that work for everyone, especially the kids. We did the same and not only have we had a ton of meaningful conversations and boisterous fun, but we also made friendships to last a lifetime.

9. **Dial down wedding worries.** Weddings are not typically baby-friendly events. Try and book a room at the venue where the baby can take a nap, or fall asleep for the night with a caregiver while you attend the wedding and can go back to the room if she needs you.

12

The Sleep Training Trap and the Myth of Self-Soothing

When Anand and Nupur Chatterjee's daughter Anaya was 4 months old, she started waking more frequently at night. The couple immediately blamed themselves: what were they doing wrong that had led to this change in her sleep pattern? Was she underfed? Should they supplement night feeds with a bottle of formula? Should they check with the doctor for any abnormalities? Was their baby a poor sleeper? These questions, and their daughter's night wakings, frequently kept them awake at night. They were unable to focus on chores and office work during the day.

Nupur and Anand could be any of us. Their dilemmas represent the dilemmas of millions of parents across the world. Most parents believe they got lucky when their baby starts doing miraculous 6–7 hour stretches at night, without waking up, by around 3 months of age. We did too! But around the 4-month mark, the celebration comes to an end. Parents go into a tizzy when their baby starts to wake every hour or two, crying out for a feed, for a walk, to be rocked.

In Anand and Nupur's home, this change in their daughter's sleep pattern caused mayhem. Anand shared the new dilemma with his coworker. His coworker suggested that the couple try sleep-training Anaya and that they would see instant results. She would be sleeping through the night without needing them to soothe and feed her back to sleep, guaranteed, the co-worker assured.

The couple was hopeful they had found the answer to their problems. So they decided to do some research on it. A quick search on it online left them a little shocked and very confused. All the websites that talked about sleep-training claimed that babies can self-soothe if we 'teach' them how to do it, which involved leaving the child to cry till the child was too tired to cry any more and slept out of exhaustion.

It is this philosophy that is at the core of the multimillion-dollar sleep-training industry that thrives particularly in Western countries. Obviously, it rattles most parents at first because it feels instinctively wrong. But parents are told by sleep trainers and, more troublingly, even close family and friends that they should 'toughen up'. That their baby 'needs' this. It's for the 'family's good'. There are even suggestions of putting on noise cancellation headphones if required to tune out the crying baby—and not give in till the child learns to settle herself.

'It just didn't sound right,' says Nupur. 'If a baby is dependent on us for everything else—feeding, diapering, bathing—how can she be capable of putting herself to sleep? Surely it's a milestone like everything else and she will get to it in her own time?'

Nupur was right. The couple eventually went with their gut feeling. When Anaya cried, their parental instinct, which was becoming stronger as they spent more time with their infant, told them that they should comfort her till she calmed down and went back to sleep. When Nupur dug deeper, she realized that what her daughter needed at this sensitive juncture was more comfort, not less. She was going through the 4-month regression (see Chapter 5, 'Your Baby's Sleep: 0 to 4 Months') and her night wakings were part of important developmental milestones as she learnt to roll over and become more aware of her surroundings.

Why Do Babies Wake Up and Cry?

Crying is a vocal sign of distress and a baby's cry elicits an immediate physiological response from an adult, what scientists call the 'caregiving instinct'. Babies go through half a dozen developmental leaps in their first year and it's a difficult time for everyone involved because babies typically need more attention, care and comforting during these phases. It is around these periods that many parents become perplexed about how to deal with broken sleep. There is a huge lack of awareness about biologically normal baby sleep and baby sleep cycles, which are typically short, which is why babies wake up frequently and need help to go back to sleep.

Before we set up GBSI, there wasn't any support group in the country that offered evidence-based peer support to parents to sail through the choppy waters of baby sleep.

It's important to understand that babies do not cry to cause you discomfort or to manipulate you. They cry because they want to express a need and the act of crying itself, numerous studies have proved, promotes nurturing and protective behaviour from parents. It is tied to their survival. The Australian Association of Infant Mental Health (AAIMH) states:

> Crying is a signal of distress or discomfort (either psychological or physical), from an infant or young child to let the caregiver know that they need help. From an evolutionary perspective, crying promotes proximity to the primary caregiver, in the interest of survival and the development of social bonds.

So, if you separate your child from you when he needs you the most, you inadvertently promote crying, essentially defeating the whole purpose of crying, which is to get help from you. The child, in turn, learns not to cry, and in effect, learns not to call for help, feeling isolated and alienated while suppressing his feelings and needs. On the other hand a child whose needs are fully taken care of, with close contact with his caregivers who respond to his every cry, will eventually stop crying simply because his developmental needs have changed and he feels taken care of.

Is My Baby a Poor Sleeper?

It is, of course, natural to feel disheartened about the intense sleep deprivation in those first few years when you don't know what's causing it. Often parents believe their children are just poor sleepers. Those who do seek support are often told to go to a sleep consultant or a sleep trainer. And just like that, you fall into the sleep-training trap that's gaining ground in India with a slew of sleep-trainers and the help of clever marketing that makes you believe you've been doing it all wrong by staying close to your baby during the night and at naptime. 'It is normal and healthy for infants and young children to wake through the night and to need attention from parents. This need not be labelled a disorder. There are no long-term health or developmental problems from babies waking at night. Responding to an infant's needs/crying will not cause a lasting "habit" but will contribute to the infant's sense of security,' explain the AAIMH's guidelines.

In reality, it is the very foundation of the parent–child connection that stands to be dismantled by the myth of sleep training. The truth is that you don't need to train your child to sleep independently to inculcate healthy sleep habits—you can do it without withholding the love, comfort, closeness and warmth that babies need at all times. It is a strong, unshakeable parental connection that is, in fact, the essential building block to deep, happy sleep. It is a connection that lasts a lifetime and spills into virtually every aspect of your life.

What Is Sleep Training?

The term 'sleep training' gets thrown about very frequently these days in parenting circles. Many parents refer to it without fully understanding what it signifies. Sleep training is essentially trying to teach a child to sleep independently—without natural and normal sleep associations that she needs to feel secure and comfortable. While sleep training, you withdraw comforting soothing techniques such as nursing, rocking, holding, walking or patting. It involves training your baby to not expect parental support at night or during naptime. It means building an ecosystem at home that separates the child's sleeping environment from her caregivers. It means expecting a baby to self-soothe by cutting the parenting cord off when it is time to sleep by saying no to feeds to fall asleep or bridge sleep cycles, by not picking up your baby when she cries to be held, by leaving your child in a crib to fend for herself. All this constitutes sleep training. In doing so, you strip the child of her basic right to parental response to her distress and the closeness all babies need till they outgrow it on their own.

Where does this expectation of wanting so desperately for our children to self-soothe before they are neurologically ready for it come from? Bestselling author of parenting books such as *The Gentle Sleep Book* and *Toddler Calm*, Sarah Ockwell-Smith, in her immensely popular essay on 'Self Settling—What Really Happens When You Teach a Baby to Self Soothe to Sleep', writes about how self-soothing is often referred to as the holy grail of baby sleep and how it is completely misguided and out of touch with the developmental needs of little children.

> 'Self-soothing' is such a misleading term. Whoever invented it has cleverly made it sound like something positive and gentle, similar to the new wave of controlled crying names such as 'controlled comforting', 'spaced soothing' and 'controlled soothing'. Clever marketing, same technique. In reality, however, you are categorically not leaving your baby to 'soothe', you are leaving them to cry, even if it is only for periods of 2 minutes at a time.

Sarah Ockwell-Smith writes that many sleep trainers push vulnerable, sleep-deprived parents to believe that it is vital to teach the skill of self-soothing to their offspring as soon as possible. That's where the slippery slope of sleep training begins. Sleep consultants often peddle studies that claim 'crying it out' has no detrimental effect on the children. However, these studies have regularly been debunked for being based on a shaky foundation, based on how the parents responded to the training, not the babies themselves. '[In] all of these previous sleep studies, no one had bothered to check the physiological stress responses of the infants, they simply made the assumption that if the infant stopped crying, the distress was gone,' says Tracy Cassels, director of Evolutionary Parenting.

Unfortunately, sleep training is a cultural norm, especially in Western countries, where paediatricians and childcare experts advise a separate room and a crib for a baby from the time he is born. Increasingly, with shorter maternity leaves and both parents working outside the home, there is huge pressure on parents to have their babies sleep independently. As Dr James McKenna puts it:

> . . . roughly speaking somewhere between 40–60 per cent of western babies are 'said' to have sleep problems to solve. My contention is that there is nothing wrong with the babies at all but the sleep model that is being culturally imposed on them which is the cause of the 'problem' and not the biology of the infant that suffers through that imposed cultural model and set of expectations it produces. From a biological point of view, one question begs answering: why or how could 40–60 per cent of otherwise healthy infants have sleep problems to solve and if this percentage is anything near the truth then the cultural and or scientific models of normal healthy sleep that underlie our cultural ideologies must reflect far more about adults than they do about babies. It also suggests that models of sleep, and our expectations and goals for parents, might actually prove to be the cause of the very sleep problems parents must try to solve!

What he is trying to say is that sleep training causes so much stress because babies are not *meant* to sleep independently, so they do not easily fall asleep on their own. So parents who sleep-train are likely to have misleading ideas about how babies should sleep and therefore have to teach their children to learn it the hard way—which causes a significant amount of distress, tears and a deep loss of connection. In Asian cultures, India in particular, sleep training is far less common and not the cultural norm, though there is a growing market for sleep trainers here too, as we mentioned before. Sometimes, however, parents end up sleep training inadvertently, without knowing they are doing it. So, we found it was important to list out the various sleep training methods (see Box 12.1) suggested for parents to equip you well to spot it from a mile away.

Box 12.1 Commonly Used Sleep Training Methods Popular with Sleep Trainers

- **Cry it out or extinction:** A baby is left to cry to sleep alone in a crib, which could take anywhere from 10 minutes to a few hours.
- **Controlled crying or the Ferber method:** Named after its inventor Richard Ferber, it bets on gradual extinction, where the child is left alone in a crib to sleep, with the parent offering some form of soothing at predetermined, increasing intervals till the child falls asleep.
- **Drowsy but awake/Pick up put down:** Here, the parent puts the child down before the child is fully asleep, and picks up the child to soothe if the baby cries and then puts the baby down again, repeating the same cycle as many times as it takes for the baby to fall asleep on his own.
- **Chair method/Camping out:** Considered less harsh than other methods, here, a caregiver 'camps' in the baby's room without offering any active soothing, and sits further and further away from the crib, till you're finally out of the door and out of sight.

- **Fading method:** Gradually phasing out sleep associations till no association is required, by offering it less each time.
- **'Gentle' sleep training:** As the sleep training industry tries to appeal to a larger market, it's becoming more crafty to woo more parents. Often there is some withdrawing of comforting soothing techniques that the child is most comfortable with, which could be nursing or walking or rocking.

Sleep trainers often lure even unwilling parents into sleep training their babies by making tall claims about the results. The carrot that is dangled in front of sleep-deprived and frustrated caregivers is that by leaving your child to cry and withholding parental contact during sleep time, your child will sleep through and never again need you at night.

In reality, this is a false, misleading claim. Most sleep-trained babies need to be trained again and again, after every sleep regression, after every illness and after every developmental leap when children typically need more attention and comforting.

Many parents who come to us have previously tried it. Some of them couldn't do it beyond a day, because the crying traumatized them, as it should. For others, who were egged on by trainers and friends to make it work, to be 'brave', reported that it worked for a few months, the child began to sleep through without needing to be soothed back to sleep by the parents, but soon after, the child fell ill or went through a developmental leap, so needed more cuddling and comforting, and then it was back to square one. So, in practice, sleep training is a recurring nightmare—for both the child and the parent. Imagine your spouse crying in the other room and calling out for you.

Wouldn't you go to him/her and offer comfort? Now imagine doing that to a baby—who is not even capable of walking, much less talking, without any defence against her parent's actions that takes away the security she seeks.

As for the claim of 'sleeping through the night'—we know that science tells us no one does. You wake up too, and do not 'sleep through the night'! Such as when you wake up to check your phone, to sip water, to use the loo, to turn the other way, to pull up your blanket closer, to cuddle with your child or partner in the middle of the night. As adults, we are neurologically equipped to soothe ourselves back to sleep with that little action that brings us some comfort, while children, till about 3–4 years of age, are not capable of doing the same thing most of the time. They are biologically built to need a caregiver to help them bridge sleep cycles, to assure them that all is well and they are safe. (See Chapter 2, 'The Baby Superpower: Sleep'). Babies and younger toddlers are simply not ready for the kind of emotional self-regulation that is required to sleep independently.

What Happens When We Sleep Train?

Coming to the consequences of sleep training, there are both short-term and long-term effects to consider. On a basic, more immediate level, leaving a child to cry is quite simply an insensitive, cruel thing to do, because a cry is a call to attention, and by not responding to this need we are abdicating a basic parental duty and crushing our parenting instincts while causing cortisol (the stress hormone) levels to rise. We are communicating to the child: 'I know you are in distress, I hear you calling out to me, but I choose not to respond.' The trust and unwavering faith that children have in us, being completely dependent on us as they are, is shattered in one stroke, and then, again and again, each time one sleep trains.

Even when the child stops calling out to the parent after being sleep trained, it doesn't mean the child has learnt emotional regulation—it just means that she has understood that no help will come. The stress levels, though, do not drop. A study examined the change in the synchrony between mothers' and infants' physiology with 25 infants in the age group of 4–10 months as part of a five-day in-patient sleep training programme, in which they learn to self-settle through the extinction of crying responses during the transition to sleep.

The researchers noted:

> On the first day of the program, mothers' and infants' cortisol levels were positively associated at initiation of nighttime sleep following a day of shared activities. Also, when infants expressed distress in response to the sleep transition, mother and infant cortisol responses were again positively associated. On the third day of the program, however, results showed that infants' physiological and behavioral responses were dissociated. They no longer expressed behavioral distress during the sleep transition but their cortisol levels were elevated. Without the infants' distress cue, mothers' cortisol levels decreased. The dissociation between infants' behavioral and physiological responses resulted in asynchrony in mothers' and infants' cortisol levels.

What this essentially means is that being left alone to sleep without comforting the baby when she asks for help by taking away biologically normal sleep associations changes the physiology, with continued heightened stress, even if they stop crying and decline to show an outwardly noticeable response. You may feel all is well once the baby stops crying after being sleep trained but that sudden quiet you experience is deceptive and misleading.

Replacing Sleep Training with Sleep Management

If you don't sleep train, does it mean your child won't sleep properly and get enough rest? Does no sleep training mean letting a child forgo a routine and sleep whenever, wherever? *Absolutely not.*

One of the joys of parenting is helping your baby create a happy and soothing relationship with sleep and build on what she is already born with—the ability to fall asleep when she feels safe and secure.

At GBSI, we guide parents through what we like to call 'sleep management'. This means:

- Nurture age-appropriate sleep associations
  Infants sleep off with nursing, rocking and gentle patting. See what works for your baby and help him sleep quickly and deeply. Stick with it for as long as it works! Remember that bedsharing with parents is what is naturally suited to babies, so cot-sleeping and sleeping in a different room can cause distress to babies and is best avoided till such a time as the child asks to sleep in a different space.

- Practise age-appropriate routines
  Babies' sleep needs to change as they grow, so keep in mind the age of the child and the awake windows best suited for

them at that stage of their development. One size does not fit all ages!

• Get your support system together
Sleep management is smoother when the whole family is involved. So get as many adults as possible to play their part. This could mean helping to create a quiet, noise-free environment (read: no to blaring television, yes to dim lighting in the evening) for the child. It could mean soothing the child to sleep, or holding the baby for naps. It could also mean giving the mother or father a break by following the same routine for the baby even if the primary caregiver isn't around.

• Connect deeply
Sleep management works best when you have a deep and close bond with your baby. If your baby trusts you, he will cooperate at bedtime too. So, remember, it's not just about sleep, it's about everything else that happens between naps too! Your overall style of parenting comes into play at sleep time. So if you tend to be autocratic and anxious as a parent, your child may resist sleep more than usual. Gentle, conscious parents have more luck promoting healthy sleep habits at home.

13

True Lies: The Reality of Baby Sleep

The many highs of parenthood are punctuated by several speed bumps, as every been-there-done-that parent will tell you. Watching your baby snooze peacefully is one of those truly special highs. But then, we know by now that your child's sleep journey isn't going to be all smooth sailing. It's our job to tell you that it is always best to be prepared for the bumps along the journey and not despair when confronted with them. Because when you despair, you look for quick solutions to what you assume is some sort of a sleep crisis. It's at this point that you may fall for misleading advice that is usually floating all over the web and in parenting circles to 'fix' your baby's wakings. Anything to get more sleep, right?

But not all advice is aligned with the complex realities of biologically appropriate child sleep. No matter where you live, you would have heard variations of well-meaning suggestions from friends, family and foes that sound like the following:

- Don't let your baby fall asleep at the breast while feeding.
- Babies will fall asleep on their own when they are tired.

- Don't let your baby sleep in your arms.
- Babies who nap less in the day sleep better at night.
- Feed your baby lots of solids at dinner so she sleeps through the night.
- Let your baby get used to sleeping with loud noises and bright lights so that he can fall asleep anywhere at any time.
- Let your baby cry, that's how they learn to sleep on their own!

These are complete myths that go against logic and sleep science and end up creating more trouble and disassociation between parent and child. Yet, they have been passed down generations, and repeated so very often by millions of people around the world, that they are routinely taken to be the ultimate truth and not questioned as often as they should.

New parents, typically, are vulnerable to these myths masquerading as the truth because they come wrapped as helpful advice from well-wishers, often legitimized by the medical community.

If you have fallen for such advice, there is no need to feel guilty. We all have, in one way or the other and you are certainly not alone. Sleep myths are popular and commonplace and have made themselves so much at home in our daily lives over many centuries that it's very hard for a new parent to separate fact from fiction, especially in the absence of awareness about why babies sleep the way they do. But these myths, when implemented, can play havoc with a child's growth and relationship with sleep.

The Long Life of Sleep Myths

The main reason sleep myths continue to thrive, despite research to prove them otherwise, is because most parents find it hard to accept that healthy, age-appropriate sleep is often not linear and doesn't look like what you imagine it would. Ask any parent what they wish for most and it's likely they will say, 'A good night's sleep!' or 'My baby sleeping through the night!' When that doesn't happen, they turn to a certain brand of sleep solutions that are actually just myths. As we have read before in this book, evolutionary biology ensures that babies and toddlers continue to wake through the night for their survival till they are neurologically ready to fall back asleep on their own without much assistance. So, an uninterrupted night's sleep is not likely to happen in the first few years of your child's life. Once you accept it, it gets easier, and your body too begins to adapt.

As a new mother or father, you are frequently given to believe that you're failing when you realize your child can't sleep without your touch or a feed or a walk and end up attributing these natural associations to something you're doing wrong, or a 'habit' that you believe you might have inadvertently let your child fall into.

To be clear, you are not failing and you haven't done anything wrong. The truth is this: babies have needs, and these 'habits' are necessary and not to be looked down upon. Babies cannot be spoilt or pampered enough. They need to be held close to a caregiver for long periods in the first few months. They need to breastfeed to sleep or be cradled and held close if the baby is on formula milk or bottle feeds. They need help in bridging sleep cycles, which means caregivers need to rock, nurse, walk or pat them back to sleep whenever they stir, till the time they are neurologically ready to go back to sleep themselves like adults. Requiring your closeness or assistance to sleep are not 'bad habits', but biologically appropriate requirements to grow and thrive. This is how children are meant to sleep. Any advice that suggests otherwise amounts to a myth perpetuated by someone who doesn't understand baby sleep science and biological needs.

In the last five years, we have come across thousands of queries on GBSI that revolve around the epidemic of misinformation that ends up hampering natural healthy sleep routines and ultimately leads to sleep deprivation for the whole family and a range of behavioural issues in decades to come. Let's examine some of the most common sleep myths that we have encountered while working as baby sleep counsellors and bust them, one by one.

Myth 1: Babies Fall Asleep on Their Own When They Are Tired

We have all seen babies who drop off to sleep in the middle of a noisy family dinner and toddlers who sleep off while watching television. Now think of a time when you slept off at an odd place at an odd time, perhaps in the middle of a family gathering or on a commute to the office. If that indeed happened, it wasn't because it was the ideal sleeping environment and the right way to sleep but because you were likely exhausted due to lack of rest at the right sleeping time. The same applies to children.

Babies drop off to sleep on their own when they are exhausted—because their body shuts down and goes into survival mode to preserve energy, fight stress and keep it running. At that moment, the body is functioning in emergency mode, and it is far from an ideal situation and not what you want to recreate every day, day after day.

It's also important to note that many babies do not fall asleep on their own even when exhausted; instead, their exhaustion manifests in other ways. The signs are extreme crankiness, looking upset and becoming hyperactive. At this point, it's hard to get them to lie down. It's hard to feed them. It's hard to help them unwind. It's hard to soothe them. It's hard to help them fall asleep. So it's vital that you manage their sleep when the time is ripe.

Myth 2: Some Babies Are Just Poor Sleepers

We have heard this often enough: 'My baby just doesn't like to sleep. She is a poor sleeper.' This isn't true. Babies are born sleepers! They love to sleep. It's what they did most of the time in the womb. But when babies are born, parents are often misled to believe sleep isn't important. Babies' crankiness is mistaken for 'being difficult' or 'attention-seeking'. Increasingly, we find that parents mistakenly try to fix this crankiness by offering a screen or by playing nursery rhymes or cartoons, which further hampers the sleep process. The crankiness is just an indication that the baby needs to sleep. As parents and caregivers, we need to pay attention to the appropriate wake spans of babies. They begin to display signs that tell you they would like to sleep. We need to be tuned in to catch those signs.

In the first few months, babies can't stay awake for more than 30–60 minutes at a stretch. This expands slowly to about 2 hours by 6 months. If they cross over from the 'tired' to the 'overtired' stage, the body starts producing cortisol, which fights sleep, making it more difficult for the baby to fall asleep and also to stay asleep.

This is what happens when you miss the 'sleep window'—described as the optimum time for babies to be put to nap, depending on their age. You are likely to miss the sleep window if you wait for them to fall asleep on their own. So we need to watch for sleep cues and take them to bed at the first signs of sleep—rubbing eyes, looking glazed and unable to focus, pulling ears. If a baby turns cranky, he has already gone from 'ready to sleep' to the 'overtired' zone.

Myth 3: Babies Should Learn to Sleep Independently

When Niharika Singhal's baby Meher was 7 months old, her aunt visited to meet the little one. Within a few hours of her arrival, the aunt noticed that Meher fell asleep while feeding on Niharika's lap, and for another nap was rocked to sleep by the nanny. She immediately told Niharika off for being a 'hyper' parent. 'Do you want this to become a habit? Just leave Meher to play. She will fall asleep when she is tired on her own. You don't have to rock her and don't let her fall asleep on your lap!'

Niharika was surprised to hear that. She had noticed that whenever she did not take Meher to nap when she rubbed her eyes and let her play on, she became so cranky that she missed her naps altogether which led to very disturbed nights and hours of crying.

As it turns out, Niharika was following her instincts and she was right. Babies cannot fall asleep independently. When babies are in the womb, cosy and warm, they spend most of their time sleeping. But when they come out into the world and are expected to fend for themselves in terms of falling asleep without the secure comfort of their parent's arms or lap, they become distressed and begin to cry.

Babies come into the world with the ability to sleep for most of the day and night because big growth happens when they sleep. But as a baby begins to feel sleepy, to make that last mile journey into dreamland they need to feel protected and reassured, a survival instinct we are all born with. As adults, we have our soothing patterns before we feel secure enough to fall asleep. It could be checking that the front door is locked, the light turned off and the room warm or cool enough. For babies, the whole soothing routine is more basic and physical, in the form of an adult's presence reassuring them that they are not going to be left alone, and it's okay to fall asleep when they're sleepy. A gentle rocking, walking, nursing acts as the perfect aid to tip the child into a restorative, deep sleep. Teaching a child to self-soothe before he is neurologically ready is the biggest con of modern-day parenting and a dangerous myth that causes immense stress to babies and their parents. Being close to a baby as he drifts off to sleep promotes connection and security.

Myth 4: Babies Sleep Better When You Remove Sleep Crutches

Most parents feel terrible guilt when their babies need a sleep association to sleep, such as nursing, holding for naps, rocking, walking, the presence of a caregiver. In reality, these natural sleep associations are age-appropriate biological needs.

One of the most common parental worries we come across in the group is this: 'My baby wakes up the moment I put him down on the bed'. This happens to almost *all* babies. It happens because babies sense separation, especially when they are infants, and they instinctively sense danger. Babies are hardwired to raise an alarm when they find themselves alone. It's how our race survived in the wild. Babies who did not raise an alarm did not live to see another day. So, if your baby wakes up when you put her down, rejoice! Your baby is displaying age-appropriate cues and is working to keep himself safe. Offer the safety he craves. That safety, for now, is in your arms.

We also tend to get thousands of queries about how to get babies to nap better in the day because most parents find their babies not sleeping enough through the day, nowhere close to the recommended number of hours. This is mainly because babies do not get the necessary sleep environment and physical contact to nap when sleepy.

As babies grow past infancy, many do not need to be held any more and are perfectly happy to sleep on when put down on the bed once in deep sleep.

But till you get to that point, it's best to know and accept that human babies need a lot of physical contact. There is a reason the first three months of life are often called 'the fourth trimester'.

At this time, the easiest way to ensure proper rest during the day is to hold your baby for her naps or at least lie down next to her.

This can sound very inconvenient. But how does it help if the baby wakes up? Sleep is very important for their development. Not to mention how insufficient sleep will lead to even more disturbed sleep and the cycle of overtiredness. Many of us have held our babies for all their naps until they were 4, 6, 8, 10 months old and beyond!

Let housework slip. Get as much help as you can. Try babywearing in an ergonomic carrier. Make yourself comfortable with water and snacks within reach. Watch some TV shows, read books, play or work on your phone. Or just snooze a bit yourself! It's very normal for babies to need this closeness. And you know what, these months will fly by. Before you know it, your child will want you to keep your nose out of her business! Hold on to them while you can.

Myth 5: Babies Sleep Better in a Cot/Separate Room

Buying a cot is one of the most sought-after activities for to-be parents who spend months looking for the perfect one, and splurge thousands on it. Many others do up the child's nursery with much pride, taken in by images in popular media and films that normalize early separation of children from their caregivers. They imagine their child moving into the nursery from the parents' room not very long after birth. One of the most pervasive myths that is catching on in India is that babies sleep better in a cot and in a separate space and all parents should aspire to pushing them into it as early as possible. But by the time your child hits 6 months, many parents realize that it is neither practical nor advisable because babies actively resist being separated from their caregivers. Do not hold this against them—they are basically doing what they are biologically designed to do for their survival!

'My worst investment!' rues Ragini Mitra. She spent close to Rs 25,000 on an imported cot from a fancy multinational store. Her son Zubin slept in it for the first four months, but only at night. 'During the day, he would be up within 20 minutes of being in the cot, but when he napped in my arms, he easily slept for an hour or two. He managed to sleep a few hours at a time in the cot during the night. After the fourth month regression, he refused to be put down in it even for a minute. He would sense he was being put down even in deep sleep and would start howling. So, after that, we only used it for storing some of his toys and happily bedshared!'

Ragini's story is a common one. Thousands of mothers we have counselled on GBSI reported that their babies woke up the moment they were put to sleep in a cot, but slept on peacefully when they bedshared with their parents. Researchers, at least the baby-friendly ones, are realizing that cot-sleeping goes against biological impulses of babies.

Even in the US, where cot-sleeping is the norm rather than the exception, as it is in India, bedsharing is a growing trend among families, reported the US-based National Public Radio (NPR). 'More moms are choosing to share a bed with their infants. Since 1993, the practice in the US has grown from about 6 per cent of parents to 24 per cent in 2015.' In India, parents have for generations slept close to their babies, for good reason. 'Human babies are contact-seekers. What they need the most is their mother's and father's bodies,' Dr James McKenna says. 'This is what's good for their physiology. This is what their survival depends on.'

In the study 'A Comparison of the Sleep–Wake Patterns of Cosleeping and Solitary-Sleeping Infants', researchers examined whether 3–15-months-old co-sleeping infants displayed differences in time spent in active versus quiet sleep, and in the number/duration of nighttime wakings when compared with solitary-sleeping infants. They found that while co-sleeping children woke more, they had shorter wakings than the ones who slept alone, suggesting that being close to their caregivers encouraged them to fall back asleep more quickly.

So, ditch that cot if your baby hates it. You do not have to move your child into a separate room if you are not comfortable with it and your child resists it. Contact sleep is what breeds connection and security. Many parents ask us: When is the right time to move the child to another bed, another room? Your child will, someday, demand his own room even without you pushing him towards it, and that's the right time to make the transition out of your family bed.

Myth 6: Babies Sleep Better Once They Start Solids

This is a truly tricky myth because it is very tempting to believe. Ask any grandparent and they will say feeding babies a heavy dinner will help them sleep through the night. It makes sense when you first hear it, but, in practice, it almost never holds true, and several medical studies have proved there is no link.

If it was true, all babies would be sleeping through the night after 6 months, because most babies are started on solids at that juncture. The reality is that solids have very little to do with sleep. Sometimes though, mothers report that baby sleep becomes more patchy once the child is introduced to solids because their gut is so immature that digestion issues are commonplace and can cause them to become more gassy and easily disturbed at night (see Chapter 6, 'Your Baby's Sleep: 5 to 7 Months').

Considerable research points to it too. In one study, 'Infant Sleep and Bedtime Cereal', researchers set out to find whether feeding infants rice cereal before bedtime promotes sleeping through the night.

One hundred six infants were randomly assigned to begin bedtime cereal feeding (1 tablespoon per ounce in a bottle) at 5 weeks or at 4 months of age. Caretakers recorded the infant's sleep from age 4 to 21 weeks for one 24-hour period per week. Sleeping through the night was defined as sleeping at least 8 consecutive hours, with the majority of time being between the hours of midnight and 6 a.m. There was no statistically significant trend or a consistent tendency of one group to have a higher proportion of sleepers than the other.

They concluded that feeding infants rice cereal in the bottle before bedtime does not appear to make much difference in their sleeping through the night.

So, there is no point in forcing your baby to eat more than she eats happily in order to make her sleep longer stretches. It will not only cause everyone immense stress, but also not work to better sleep. Imagine how you feel after a terribly heavy dinner. Your baby would feel highly uncomfortable too and unlikely to be able to sleep peacefully.

Myth 7: You Can Train a Baby to Sleep through the Night

All humans wake at the end of a sleep cycle. As adults, we are able to roll over and go back to sleep, starting a new sleep cycle. Babies develop this skill closer to 2–3 years of age. By about 3–4 years, you will notice your child will not need your help to go back to sleep, though she will prefer to sleep with you and be comforted by having her parents next to her.

But until this important milestone is reached, they need our help to transition cycles. This is a developmental milestone like walking or talking and cannot be rushed. Some sleep trainers tout the benefits of a baby sleeping 'uninterrupted', but, as you can see, nobody sleeps uninterrupted, including adults. Babies can get ample and fairly continuous sleep with some parental input.

The idea that one should put the baby down 'drowsy but awake' and hence, 'break sleep associations' or 'teach the baby to sleep on her own' and 'sleep through the night' is a pet concept of most sleep trainers, but several sleep experts absolutely dismiss the entire idea.

Firstly, very few babies actually accept the whole 'drowsy but awake' method without protest and some amount of crying. Secondly, even if your baby accepts it and manages to complete the falling asleep process on her own, there is no guarantee that she will wake less frequently, or that not having a parent-dependent sleep association means they can bridge sleep cycles on their own and technically sleep through the night.

Breaking sleep associations is a form of sleep training. It's basically trying to teach a baby to 'self-settle', which is unscientific as babies don't have that brain capacity at all. In fact, the easiest way for the baby and parent to get enough rest is to co-sleep and nurse lying down. Anything else just creates more stress for both.

Myth 8: Weaning from the Breast Leads to Sleeping through the Night

Mothers often decide to wean from the breast, particularly at night, because they are told it will help the child sleep on their own and eliminate nightwakings.

Unfortunately, this often backfires and makes things even more chaotic for the mother, especially during regressions when babies and toddlers need more comforting at night. For one, breastmilk is the primary source of nutrition in the first year and feeds should not be restricted. Babies need to feed even out of hunger and for nutrition at night. So, trying to 'break' this 'association' should definitely not be attempted in the first year.

Two, breastfeeding assists sleep, rather than hamper sleep, as is often believed. The sleep-inducing hormone melatonin is passed to babies through breastfeeding, with higher levels in nighttime breast milk. Isn't that amazing?

Breastfeeding is indeed the most natural, normal, convenient and effective way to make your baby sleep well into toddlerhood.

The easiest way to handle the transitions between cycles, if you are indeed breastfeeding, is through breastfeeding, because it is designed to aid sleep. One can also rock or walk or pat if breastfeeding is not an option. It is possible for the mother to nurse to sleep and the father or another caregiver to use another method. Babies adapt well to multiple methods of soothing from multiple caregivers.

It's natural for older toddlers too to feed to sleep and wake up at night and go back to sleep by nursing. They don't wake up to feed, as is often misunderstood; they wake up because their brain is still immature and they need help to transition to the next sleep cycle, and feeding acts as a natural sleep aid. So even if you wean a toddler from the breast, he is likely to continue to wake up and need other ways to fall asleep. So before you wean, it's best to weigh your options by being aware of the science behind the cause of your child's wakings. Empowered and aware parents always make better choices.

Myth 9: Formula Feeds Make Babies Sleep Longer

Although urban legend claims formula-fed babies sleep longer and deeper, there is varying scientific evidence on this. Some studies that have compared how breastfed and formula-fed babies sleep show a statistically significant difference. But anecdotal evidence from parents around us gives varying reports. Many formula-feeding parents are equally sleep deprived and exhausted. Some do testify to longer stretches of sleep. However, there are several other parenting practices that are not accounted for in these cases and so it is difficult to draw any solid conclusions.

Formula is heavier than breastmilk and takes longer to digest. While this can lead to some longer stretches of sleep in the newborn stage when baby tummies are really very small, the heaviness of formula can also cause stomach troubles like gas which can disturb sleep. Furthermore, the link between a full stomach and long hours of sleep is not strong. If it was, the introduction of solids would ensure breastfed babies too slept longer hours, which doesn't happen.

Some studies have shown that breastfed babies wake more easily from active sleep. While this makes them more prone to nightwakings, it is also what contributes to the lower risk of SIDS recorded amongst breastfed babies, according to experts.

And here is the irony: while breastfed babies may be waking more, breastfeeding mums report more sleep. Nursing mothers benefit from high levels of sleep-inducing hormones like prolactin, experience more than double the normal duration of nocturnal slow wave sleep, and may be able to sleep during nighttime feeds, if they bedshare and nurse lying down. Formula feeding parents report that preparing a bottle is far more disruptive, long-winded and that they find it harder to go back to sleep.

Babies sleep longer hours/sleep through the night when they are developmentally ready for it. They wake for several reasons at night—at the end of sleep cycles or due to some internal or external factor that they are incapable of regulating on their own. No single factor, like milk source, can override this developmental trajectory.

14

Keeping Them Cosy: The Truth about Sleep Associations and Why Babies Need Them

Human beings are creatures of habit. Especially when it comes to rituals around sleep, night after night, we crave to go back to comforting associations that make us feel secure and relaxed as we close our eyes and drop off to sleep.

These are associations we have inculcated over time that help us stay asleep, often unconsciously. They vary from person to person depending on our personalities and individual needs. Think of your own sleep rituals. What does it take for you to wind down and close your eyes? A favourite pair of pyjamas, an old T-shirt, a particular side of the bed? Do you sleep better on a certain kind of mattress and pillow? Do you need a quiet and dark room? A relaxing book? Music? A cool room? Often, it's a combination of things that lull you to sleep. As you would have noticed by now, your child needs a sleep ritual too. When they are infants, just a quick feed at the breast or a bottle and the comfort of your arms is enough for them to plop off to sleep. As they grow, they need a more elaborate winding-down routine. Here's a little experiment. Write down the associations that help you sleep. Then make another list of the associations your child needs to sleep.

You'll see that babies and adults are not all that different when it comes to sleep. Of course, babies need to sleep a lot more, but we all need some kind of associations and aids to signal it is time for bed. The associations help us create a predictable pattern that acts as a well-oiled machine as natural light dims, the sky darkens, night falls and our bodies feel the weight of the day. The process of winding up work, clearing up after dinner and getting ready for bed is so routine that we don't really think about it any more unless there is a major disruption. But children need help with the same process because they are dependent on us to create sleep rituals.

You'll find that babies under the age of 3 years often need active forms of soothing to go to sleep as opposed to older children and adults, who can be easily comforted by passive sleep aids.

What Are Active Forms of Soothing?

Nursing, holding, rocking or walking to sleep constitute active soothing, that require some effort on the part of the soother. These are methods of soothing that babies respond to keenly. They have a very high success rate because these are instinctive, natural, biologically appropriate sleep aids that lull them to sleep within minutes (when done in keeping with an age-appropriate routine and a soothing sleep environment). Human beings are wired to need reassurances, both internal and external, and your baby no doubt needs them too, especially as she falls asleep. Children need to know they are safe, not alone and taken care of.

However, sleep associations are also at the centre of one of the biggest sleep myths perpetuated by the sleep training industry worldwide that claims they are a 'sleep crutch' or a 'sleep prop'.

Cultural conditioning that seeks to separate children from parents at an early stage will have you believe that nursing, holding, walking or rocking children fall under 'negative' sleep associations. Parents are routinely chastised for allowing their babies to form these 'habits'. The truth is that, as babies grow, they learn to sleep in different ways *on their own*—it need not be hurried or taught in any way. Habits and needs change with time.

So, dear parent, we cannot stress enough that these fears of creating 'bad habits' are unfounded and unnecessary. We do, however, acknowledge that there is a tremendous amount of confusion among parents on the sleep aids that are biologically appropriate and the ones that are not. It can often be very baffling, especially as a new parent, because there is a barrage of advice coming from numerous quarters on what's right and what's not. In this chapter, we will discuss *how to create necessary and healthy sleep associations*, such as a dark, soothing room and the comfort of a caregiver close by, while clearing the air on sleep aids such as pacifiers, swaddling, loveys and white noise that parents often wonder about.

The Sleep Aids Your Baby Needs

Nursing to sleep

It's not a coincidence that most babies fall asleep while nursing. It's nature's way of aiding nutrition, sleep and, consequently, early child development. Food and sleep are the biggest drivers of child growth and nursing fuels them both. But far too often you will find people discouraging mothers from letting their children fall asleep at the breast. The world's leading authority on mother-infant co-sleeping, Dr James McKenna, explains it best: breast-sleeping is biologically normal. This essentially means that it is natural for a child to fall asleep at the breast. Breastmilk acts as a sleep aid, releasing the hormone prolactin that calms both mother and child and makes them sleepy. Breastmilk made at night, meanwhile, also contains melatonin, passing on to the baby and helping him fall asleep. So bed-sharing while offering free access to your child to feed whenever he stirs at night—what McKenna calls breast-sleeping—is really the most biologically appropriate sleep association.

As we have discussed earlier (in chapter 13, 'True Lies: The Reality of Baby Sleep'), no-one really sleeps through the night. All humans wake at the end of a sleep cycle. The easiest way to handle the transitions between cycles for babies is through breastfeeding, unless of course you are a bottle-feeding parent. In which case, a bottle of milk followed by walking or rocking should work.

But for those who do breastfeed, it's important to know that breastmilk is the primary source of nutrition in the first year and feeds should not be restricted. Babies need to feed even out of hunger and for nutrition at night. So, trying to 'break' this association should definitely not be attempted in the first year.

In fact, breastfeeding is the most natural, normal, convenient and effective way to make your baby sleep well into toddlerhood.

Often, mothers are repeatedly advised to unlatch the baby when drowsy and let him fall asleep without further assistance. Very few babies actually accept the whole 'drowsy but awake' thing without protest and some amount of crying. To actively prevent a baby from falling asleep at the breast is counter-intuitive, since the very act of feeding assists sleep in the most organic way.

We believe that the most natural, and often the easiest, way for the baby and parent to get enough rest is to co-sleep and nurse lying down, which becomes a wonderful sleep bond and offers endless comfort and nourishment for the baby. Many parents worry that nursing lying down causes ear infections—this is simply not true. This is because babies' positions do not change when they feed. They are anyway lying down, propped up with your arm, whether you feed sitting up or lying down. It's your position that changes! So, it has no connection with ear infections, which happen due to a variety of reasons. Breastfed children do not require help with burping either beyond the first few weeks/months, depending on the child's comfort level. If the child has no reflux issues, is sleeping fine after the feed and does not spit up, you don't need to get up and burp the baby. Bottle feeding on the other hand can be tricky and children must be elevated while feeding, any dribble wiped off and burped after the feed. Bottle-feeding, bedsharing and cuddling after the feed goes a long way in creating a helpful sleep association.

Nursing also offers the sucking reflex, which acts as a calming mechanism for babies. It's important to note that thumb-sucking, especially in infants, is a developmental phase and usually nothing to worry about. Studies have shown that thumb-sucking is more common amongst bottle-fed infants, those who are fed on a schedule versus on cue or have been left alone to fall asleep. It is a primitive self-soothing reflex. Constant thumb-sucking, though, may cause dental issues. Most children outgrow it by 2 years of age. If it continues post the second-year mark, you might need to intervene and replace it with other ways of soothing, such as increased cuddles, nursing and holding.

Cuddling and holding

When Neha's son was an infant, she held him for naps on her lap as she read book after book. Nobody told her to do it. She had no dearth of househelp. But it felt normal and natural and her son also slept peacefully this way. But a neighbour who dropped by to congratulate her on a new baby thought this was a very odd thing to do. 'He will get used to it and then never sleep on the bed!' she exclaimed. 'Don't create bad habits!' she warned. At the time, Neha had read very little on parenting and certainly wasn't aware of the science behind baby sleep. But she did know it in her bones that she wasn't doing anything wrong. Her son had no trouble sleeping beautifully on the bed too, though he would wake at the end of a 20–30-minute sleep cycle. So, holding him felt right. He slept longer and deeper.

When we began to explore how babies sleep and why they sleep the way they sleep, we realized it felt right to hold our babies as they napped because we are biologically designed to keep our babies close—while awake as well as asleep. As they grow, they begin to offer signs of wanting independence as they start to crawl, walk, run. But in the first few months, holding is everything. Your arms are their home.

Walking and rocking

Walking and rocking can seem labour-intensive when compared to breastfeeding to sleep. But these are very effective methods that can be used by mothers who do not breastfeed, by fathers or other caregivers. Babies also go through phases when they prefer walking or rocking instead of nursing. Often, you may need to work out a combination of a couple of methods, such as nursing followed by walking or rocking. If you're walking to sleep, make sure you are doing it in a dark and quiet room. If your baby prefers to sleep off while listening to soothing music, you can switch on your favourite playlist as you walk or rock as well. Rocking can work in two ways: on your lap, or with your legs outstretched, cradling the baby in the middle. Pro tip: Try to get a rocking chair for yourself. It may help in rocking the baby to sleep in the first year or two.

Music or white noise

When Neha's son was 4 months old and going through the 4th-month regression, nothing seemed to help him sleep—not nursing, not walking nor rocking. But one day, her husband switched on Indian classical music, and voila! he immediately quietened down and slept off within 10 minutes. Talking to parents across the world, she discovered they weren't alone. Music can do wonders for babies, especially during regressions or if your baby is overtired, overstimulated and cranky. It centres them and offers a kind of meditation. The trick is to find the kind of music that works for your baby. Avoid loud, fast-paced music, and try gentle genres, like light pop or instrumental sounds. Try your favourites and see what clicks with your child. Some children do become overstimulated with music so you want to avoid it if it doesn't work. White noise, meanwhile, can be a miracle worker to aid sleep. White noise refers to sounds that mask ambient sounds streaming in from outside—like the sound of water flowing through a forest with birds chirping in the background. Even a slightly noisy fan or air purifier works well as white noise. If white noise works for your child, it might be worth investing in a white noise machine. You can also make do with a white noise app on your phone, or stream white noise via YouTube. It's important to note that while playing music or white noise, keep the baby away from any screen. Screens are not recommended for kids under 2, and even after that, if it is being offered, it should ideally be for a very limited time and definitely not at least 2 hours before sleep time.

Sleep Aids You Don't Need

Swaddling

Swaddling means to wrap the child up in a soft cloth to create a cocoon effect similar to the womb. Traditionally, swaddling was done to reduce the Moro reflex, which is an uncontrolled movement of limbs, twitching of the body, common to infants, which results in waking. Even though a swaddle is meant to create a cosy sleep environment, it cannot replace physical contact with the parent and is an artificial sleep aid. So it often doesn't work as babies resist it after the first few days or weeks of birth. Hundreds of queries on GBSI revolve around the issue of swaddling. 'My baby hates to be swaddled, but if he/she wakes up when not swaddled—what should I do?'

The answer is simple. Ditch the swaddle, or try a loose swaddle which leaves the hands free and space for movement of the legs. A tight swaddle is not recommended any more as there is now enough data that proves that restrictive swaddling is associated with hip and joint issues in babies. A much better alternative is a sleep bag/sleep sack for babies that allows some movement.

Swaddling also hinders natural movement of the body. For example, babies use their hands to soothe themselves, but swaddling inhibits this movement, making them cry out in displeasure and resist or throw off the cloth. Swaddling can also mask hunger cues. If your baby wakes up due to startling, it's best to hold her in your arms so she can quickly go back to sleep, feeling assured to find herself cradled safely.

Rockers and swings

A swing or 'jhula' is a traditional feature in many Indian homes as it is seen as a convenient sleep aid. Most of our mothers and grandmothers tend to recommend it as the go-to soothing method for babies. However, rockers and swings are not recommended any longer as they pose a major safety risk especially when babies start to turn over. They run the risk of falling out. Another big hazard is a suffocation risk as it tends to block air flow. Some newborns do seem to sleep unnaturally long stretches in them (most likely due to the blocked air flow), which can affect the breastfeeding relationship as they do not show hunger cues and do not wake to feed often enough. It is also difficult to wean babies off the jhula as they grow older, which leads to more sleeplessness and exhaustion for the caregivers, who would need to keep the swing moving all night long. In her professional practice, dozens of parents have come to Himani with a 7 or 8 month old who is no longer sleeping comfortably in a swing but is also unable to sleep without it. Alternatively, the baby is sleeping long stretches in the swing but still seems permanently overtired because the sleep is not restorative. The baby has no other sleep association and the parents are not accustomed to the rhythm of nursing, rocking, holding, bedsharing either. This creates a Catch-22 situation where the baby cannot sleep comfortably in the swing but cannot sleep without it either. A month or more of utter chaos and exhaustion ensues while parents try to set other soothing practices in place. Instead of using a swing, practise bed-sharing, breast-sleeping and holding for naps—it will make life much easier for everyone involved.

Box 14.1 The Importance of the Right Sleep Environment as a Sleep Aid

Sleep patterns are determined by a complex interplay between genetic, behavioural, environmental and social factors. Increasingly, studies find that adults and children sleep less than the recommended number of hours.

How can we ensure more sleep?

Apart from co-sleeping, there are various aspects to the baby's sleep environment that need to be addressed to ensure that the baby is set up for as peaceful a nap as possible:

1. Absence of light in any form, including night lights, phone screens, etc.
2. A quiet room away from the hustle and bustle of the house.
3. Optimal room temperature ensuring that it's neither too hot nor too cold. 22–24°C is usually comfortable enough.
4. Bedding that has no loose sheets.
5. Comfortable clothing that doesn't overheat the baby nor is overly restrictive.

Bottles

Bottles can be very convenient in the first year of birth if the mother needs to step out of the home. It helps alternative caregivers feed the child. However, if your baby needs a bottle to fall asleep, it's time to revisit the whole sleep ritual. It's best to not use bottles as a sleep aid because it is artificial and can quickly become an association that hampers your child's development in more ways than one. One way to break the association is to burp the baby once the child finishes feeding from a bottle, and soothe her to sleep by rocking or walking. It's also important to note that bottles must be weaned after the age of 1 year, as bottle-feeding can increase chances of cavities due to the milk pooling around the baby's mouth, making it a dental hazard. This doesn't happen when a child breastfeeds, but is a risk with bottle-feeding. When you're trying to wean from a bottle, try to replace the soothing by offering active soothing such as holding, walking or rocking.

Cots and cribs

Raise your hand if you—before your child's entry into your home—believed that buying the best-looking cot would help your baby sleep quick and easy. Now raise your hand if your child woke up wailing the minute you put him down in that cot. If you are nodding furiously, you are not alone! Most parents spend months looking for the prettiest cot in town only to be greatly disappointed that their child does not like it as much as they did. Within months of the child's birth, reality strikes. This is because there is a biological reason behind it. *Cots do not necessarily aid sleep.*

Babies may do well in a crib the first few months at night. But it's very common for babies to start resisting cots after the 4-month-, 8-month- or the 12-month regressions. It's not linked to the regression as much as growing developmental awareness of being separated from their caregivers. At that point, when the baby starts to resist it, you can take a call on whether you'd like to persist, gently, or abandon it altogether. Babies need security and connection to be able to sleep, and cots and cribs come in the way of that. Your magic word here is bedsharing. The sleep aid your child needs is to be next to you on your family bed. Pro tip: Instead of splurging on an imported cot, go for a king-size family bed that's got enough room for everyone to snuggle. Hundreds of parents report that their cots now make a neat (though expensive) home for laundry and soft toys. Our cots were definitely useful in the first few months. After the 4-month regression though, they sat neglected in a corner, except on occasion when we popped the baby in to keep him or her safe if we were alone at home and needed to use the washroom/answer the door or when we used it as an occasional playpen.

Pacifiers and soft objects like loveys

'My baby is using me as a pacifier! What should I do?' is a common query on GBSI. Ironically, pacifiers were invented sometime in the early 1900s, nicknamed Baby Comforter, built to mimic a nipple. In the first 6 months of a baby's life, sucking forms a huge part of their development that comes from breastfeeding. When babies suckle, they are not only deriving nutrition, but also soothing themselves at the breast. 'Suckling allows learning and synchronicity of several functions that have an important morphogenetic role in the harmonious development of the craniofacial complex of the child,' found a study.

Pacifiers have become controversial these days as experts warn that introducing them too early can severely disrupt the breastfeeding relationship, cause nipple confusion and supply issues. Introducing them later, after the first few months, can become a challenge too, as it is hard to wean off from them, and they can become a source of infection very quickly, as they tend to fall off from the baby's mouth.

Add to that, several studies have found a correlation between the ear infection Otitis Media and pacifier use by a backflow from the nasopharynx to the Eustachian tube. In one study, the children who did not use a pacifier continuously had 33 per cent fewer episodes of the ear infection than the children who did. Prolonged pacifier use can cause misalignment of the teeth. What pacifiers offer is essentially prolonged non-nutritive sucking, which can lead to speech abnormalities too. 'The greater the longevity and duration of pacifier use, the greater the potential for harmful results,' noted one study.

Pacifiers can be useful for infants who have gone through specific minor surgeries, or to strengthen the suck–swallow reflex for premature infants on recommendation by a lactation consultant in conjunction with breastfeeding. But, for others, especially breastfeeding children, it should be introduced with caution, if at all, and weaned off before 6 months, after which risks of infection increase. If used, the pacifier needs to be regularly sterilized and replaced when worn out.

Soft objects, such as loveys, are commonly used in Western countries as a way to encourage self-soothing and a way to replace the caregiver's presence, especially among toddlers and pre-schoolers. Some cultures have a greater dependence on it than others. In many non-Western cultures, for example, loveys are not commonplace because there is frequent physical contact between children and a caregiver, most often the mother, which eliminates any need for an artificial object.

So, should you introduce a lovey?

No loveys for babies under 12 months as they can pose a suffocation risk. After that, you may see if your child takes to one. Most children will not respond to it with much enthusiasm. But you may notice, around age 2–3 years, that your child shows an inclination to take her favourite toy to bed with her. Though no object can replace the warmth and security of a parent or a close caregiver.

Box 14.2 How Did Previous Generations Do It?

Parents are often puzzled about why their child's sleep can seem so hard to navigate. Our parents didn't spend so much time worrying about sleep. And they have so many children! How did they do it? One way to answer this is to look at the average family size and living setup. Living in a joint family afforded them many hands to help. Sleep aids were easier to come by: cousins and siblings, aunts and uncles, grandmothers and grandfathers were frequently around to rock or hold babies to sleep. Research on sleep and access to information was scant. Not many bothered about how much their child was sleeping. Crankiness and behavioural problems were put down to being a part and parcel of growing up. They had limited resources, tight budgets and other priorities. Sleep was simply not a top concern. It was a different time. Traditional jhulas were commonplace. They are now considered a suffocation risk. It wasn't unusual to offer babies a few drops of sleep-including herbal concoctions, gripe water (containing alcohol) and other medications to get them to fall asleep quickly. None of these are recommended any more by medical professionals as they are known to cause long-term harm.

15

Sleep for Siblings

The arrival of a sibling is a major life event for a toddler or pre-schooler. While we may view it as the normal course of things (almost everyone has more than one kid, right!), it is far from ordinary for our first child, especially if that child is under 4 years old. Scientists have theorized that natural birth spacing in prehistoric times would have been three to four years. Since breastfeeding suppresses ovulation and mothers breastfed on demand for at least two years, there is some credence to the idea that human children have evolved to thrive with a three to four year spacing between siblings. Since human children also need a lot of carrying, care and parental input in the early years, it stands to reason that having the undivided attention of parents in the early years would lead to some healthy outcomes. Once a child is 3.5 to 4 years old, sleeping mostly through the night, capable of some amount of reasoning and emotional self-regulation, no longer in diapers and perhaps going to school, a new entrant in the family is easier for the child and the parents to manage.

Of course, an ideal gap between siblings in modern society (or even the need for a sibling at all) can be debated until the cows come home, and there is no 'correct' answer. There may be a whole host of other reasons that make it prudent to have children in quick succession. Babies are not always strictly planned either. It is reasonable to say, however, that the arrival of a sibling is a tricky affair, especially if the older one is under 4 years old. There are some factors to consider and plan for, one of which is definitely sleep.

The Younger Sibling's Sleep

As we know, newborns need a lot of contact and soothing to sleep. For our firstborns, we may have completely devoted ourselves to their sleep and nursing needs. Our baby may have barely left our arms in those early weeks. Our second baby doesn't know she is our second baby and actually needs exactly the same thing. The tragedy is that we can't give them the same thing because we have an older one to take care of as well.

Himani had her second daughter when her first was just under two-and-a-half years old. Here is how she suggests we can make this situation easier for the baby:

1. **Arrange help**

   If you have family around or if you can hire a caregiver, please ask for help without holding back. This is one time in your life that you really need it. Himani ensured that she was never alone at home with her two kids. Either her husband or a grandparent or a caregiver was with her at all times. In the early days, she would nurse the baby and then, for most naps, someone else would hold her to ensure the baby slept long stretches while Himani tended to her toddler. In the newborn phase, little babies will accept any loving human. As she grew older and needed specifically her mother for her naps, the other adult could help take care of the older one.

2. Babywear

Use a wrap or a ring sling or a newborn-appropriate buckled carrier and try to get your baby used to sleeping in it. Watch videos or ask for the help of a baby-wearing educator to ensure you are wearing the baby correctly to maximize your chances of success.

3. Merge naps

If your older one is still napping, try to make them nap around the same time so that you can lie between them and manage them both.

4. Use a video baby monitor

Himani considers this her most prized possession since the birth of her first child, allowing her to step out during naps and after bedtime while catching the first signs of a stir, enabling her to rush back in to nurse or cuddle the baby back to sleep. After the birth of the second, it became all the more valuable because it enabled her to be with one child while the other napped.

5. Create a safe space outside the home for the older one

Like a daycare or a preschool or a grandparent's home. The idea is not to force the older one to be out of the house. The space should always be gentle, emotionally safe and something the older one goes to happily. This outing gives the mother three to four hours to devote to the newborn to bond in an undistracted and exclusive way.

6. **Make an activity box**

   It's a good idea to prepare this while you are pregnant and then refresh it once a month. Put aside 21–28 activities, including some sensory items—like straws, stickers, bubble wrap, sensory jars—in a large box. Designate a smaller box for daily use. Every day, dump three or four new activities into the smaller box and produce this to your toddler when you need to nurse your baby or rock to sleep and need to keep your toddler busy for a while. Change the activities every day and rotate on a weekly basis so that they remain fresh for your toddler.

7. **Develop a reading habit and invest in books**

   Reading picture books with your toddler can be a lifesaver. It is a wonderful activity to do while you are nursing your newborn or holding for naps. Invest in a mini-library of books and keep changing the stack of books readily at hand.

8. **Don't let big sis or big bro wake the baby**

   And yet, constantly shouting 'don't wake the baby!' is going to be counterproductive. Toddlers cannot control their impulses, and constantly being told off can make the older sibling resent the baby. Toddlers also like to test limits and may consciously do exactly the opposite of what we ask them to. It's a better idea to plan ahead and keep the toddler engrossed in another activity while the baby is sleeping.

9. **Hang in there**

   Babies move to three naps at 6 months and two naps at 8 months. It becomes much easier to handle once they have a more or less predictable schedule.

Box 15.1 Should You Let Your Older One Watch TV While You Handle the Baby?

The general recommendation around screen time is *zero screen* before the age of 2 years, and a maximum of 1 hour (built up slowly) up till the age of 5 years. The detrimental effects of screen time are numerous, ranging from slowing down language development to affecting attention spans and sleep. If you decide to allow, say, 30 minutes of TV for your two-and-a-half year old, use it strategically and try to not exceed the allowance you have decided upon. It's tempting to use television as a babysitter, but we would encourage you to use the strategies we have suggested above instead of relying heavily on screens.

The Older Sibling's Sleep

The arrival of a new sibling is a tumultuous time for a toddler. Even though a toddler may appear (and may also genuinely feel) very excited, the change in the family's dynamics usually comes as a shock. Although a toddler may be very loving and caring to the baby, coping with the parents' divided attention is often too much for their primitive brains. Toddlers often display challenging behaviour soon after the arrival of a sibling. The logistical challenges in sleep management are exacerbated by the emotional turmoil. So, there are two aspects to handling your older one. Firstly, the management of her actual sleep. Secondly, the management of her emotional state.

Preparation during Pregnancy

Himani's older one had self-weaned during her pregnancy and her sleep had gone for a massive toss as a result. They had several active nightwakings during the pregnancy, where Himani or her husband had to walk her (or drive her, all else failing). Many toddlers do self-wean when the mother is pregnant due to a drop in supply and change in the taste of the milk as it converts into colostrum for the newborn baby, but many do not. There is usually no need to wean your toddler if you are pregnant, as long as you have a healthy, no-risk pregnancy. Please do consult a breastfeeding-friendly gynaecologist and, if needed, a qualified lactation consultant as well. There are many benefits to nursing through a pregnancy and thereafter tandem-feeding, difficult though it sounds. Mothers also report less emotional trauma to the older sibling if he or she is still nursing when the younger one arrives.

If the mother is the primary sleep caregiver for the firstborn, it is a good idea to make the toddler less dependent on the mother in the last months of pregnancy. This does not mean an abrupt withdrawal of the mother as that would just traumatize the baby, but a very gradual and gentle involvement of the father or alternate caregiver. Like with all things related to baby sleep, it is usually best to cross each bridge when you come to it; trying to form 'habits' usually does not work and months that would otherwise be calm and secure become unstable in anticipation of some future uncertainty. So, it is important to maintain a balance between involving the father and allowing the child to have her mother for as long as possible. As clinical psychologist Dr Laura Markham says, 'It's important to recognise that your child does not see her parents as interchangeable. If she loses

Mom to the new baby, she'll grieve and resent the baby—even if she gets exclusive rights to Dad. So, it's important that each parent get time with each child.'

If the toddler has been primarily nursing to sleep, the father can use methods like walking a baby to sleep with music, or babywearing or, as a last resort, taking the baby for a drive in a car as methods to soothe the little one to sleep.

During Himani's second pregnancy, she and her husband tried to make their daughter less dependent on her at night and to nudge her to turn to her father for soothing. This worked to an extent but not entirely. Although she had always been extremely attached to her father, sleep was associated almost entirely with her mother. The best that they could achieve was that her toddler accepted her father approximately three out of ten times and they considered this a win!

Himani and her husband were also extremely concerned about what would happen to their tot for the one or two nights that she would be in the hospital for the delivery. Their older one had never slept a single night without her mother. They did a few practice naps at her grandmother's house but were still not sure how night sleep would go. 'I prayed and prayed that my delivery would be during the day so that my husband could reach my older one for the night,' Himani says. 'I was more worried about my older one's night sleep than my labour!'

Fortunately for them, their second one was a '9 to 5' baby. They reached the hospital at 9 a.m. and the baby was out at 4.30 p.m. The firstborn was with her grandmother and a caregiver for her nap and her father reached her before bedtime, while Himani's mother stayed with her in the hospital with the newborn. This was their toddler's first ever night without her mother and she handled it like a champ! It's true that babies do surprise you. She slept just fine with her father. Himani believes that she would have risen to the occasion even if she'd had to stay with only her grandmother that night.

Things were not so easy in the days, weeks and months that followed. Himani's toddler needed her at night. There were nights when she cried and Himani cried even more. Himani tried her best to juggle both the babies at night, but perfection was impossible. It took a few weeks for her to completely attach herself to her father for night sleep but it did happen.

The Older Sibling's Nap

The naps of the older sibling also need proper attending to. If only one parent is available, the best would be to arrange help to tend to the newborn while the parent soothes the older one to sleep. Other options are breastfeeding the newborn while lying next to the toddler or making the toddler sleep once the newborn is asleep.

Possible Sleeping Arrangements

There are many sleeping arrangements for co-sleeping families with two kids, and there is no one answer for this. You will need to figure out what works for you by trial and error. Different things may work for different families and at different times. You can explore:

- The mother sleeping in between the newborn and toddler, with the father on the other side of the toddler.
- The newborn in a sidecar crib or co-sleeper, with the toddler in between the parents.

- The father and older child in one room, the mother and younger child in another room so that the children do not wake each other at night.
- Everyone in one room until one of the children wakes at night, at which point one parent and one child leave to go to another room.

Some siblings manage to sleep together without disturbing each other and some do not. You will need to see what works for you. You can try white noise as a way of drowning out either child's noises.

Box 15.2 Should You Shift the Older Sibling to His Own Room?

If your child has been co-sleeping so far, it is not a good idea to shift him to a separate room either before or after the baby's arrival. Shifting him too close to the baby's arrival or immediately after can be traumatic for the child and lead to resentment towards the baby. It can also lead to a lot of unnecessary struggles between the parents and the child, adding to your already high stress levels. Choose your battles! It is very reassuring to your toddler to have one parent or both with him through the night at an otherwise unstable time.

Bedtime Routines

Bedtime routines are unlikely to be at the same time as each child will have her individual schedule based on awake windows and circadian rhythms (or lack thereof!). The ideal scenario—and honestly, the only smooth one—is for one parent to handle one bedtime routine while the other parent takes care of the other child. Both parents should go out of their way to ensure that this is possible. If it is absolutely impossible, then it is best to brace for some chaos. The mother can babywear the newborn while taking the toddler through his bedtime routine of changing into pyjamas and brushing his teeth. The newborn can nurse or play in an activity gym while the mother reads to the toddler. Then, if the toddler can be cuddled to sleep, the best way to do this would be to nurse the newborn alongside. If the toddler needs to be walked to sleep, it is going to be a tricky affair. The only way it would be possible is for the younger sibling to be asleep at the time, which may lead to some overtiredness in case the toddler has to wait.

The Role of the Father

If the father is not already an equal caregiver before the arrival of a second child, it is definitely time to step up when another baby joins the family. The father's role kicks in during pregnancy itself, when he should work on shifting the older one's care to himself—from spending quality time during the day to handling the bedtime routine to soothing the child to sleep for naps and at night to handling night wakings. If the father works outside the home, he can pitch in as much as possible after work, at night and on weekends.

After the arrival of the new baby, it is very important for the father to not only take over the toddler's care, and work on making the transition as emotionally seamless as possible for her, but also to participate equally in the newborn's care so that the toddler gets precious time with her mother. Since paternity leave is not recognized in India, it is a good idea to use as much regular leave as possible during this time and to also discuss your needs with your manager.

Handling Emotions

The arrival of a sibling is a highly emotional time for the family. No matter how much one prepares, it's a tornado when it happens. For the post-partum mother who is exhausted and high on hormones, it's a time of immense grief, guilt and heartache. For the father, it's a time of exhaustion and immense strain because, in many cases, this is the time when the father becomes the primary caregiver for the older child. But, more than anything, the emotional state of the older sibling needs attending to. While a comprehensive explanation on this subject will require a whole other book, here are the main pointers:

1. Prepare the older sibling for the baby's arrival during pregnancy—read books about sibling arrival, let the baby talk to your belly, involve your firstborn in choosing the name and in doing up the baby's space.
2. Manage the first meeting between the older and younger sibling. Have the father or someone else hold the baby when they first meet. Make the older child the centre of the event. Arrange a small and meaningful 'gift' from the baby to the older child.
3. Get your older one a doll to care for the way you care for the baby.
4. Involve your older one in caring for the baby, like getting you diapers, putting cream on the baby, showing baby toys, singing to the baby, etc.

5. If your older child is traumatized by your nursing the younger one due to feelings of jealousy and proprietorship, talk to her about it, explain that breastmilk is baby's food, but, until she/he is okay with it and if you have another adult around, just leave the room to nurse. It's not worth the trauma. Save your older one the pain and work on it slowly.

6. Help your older one express his feelings. Use phrases like 'It can be very hard to be an older brother' and 'You didn't ask for a baby and now you feel so strange to have a little baby in the house' and 'It's okay to be sad'.

7. Use tools like an 'empathy book', a book where you draw out, page by page, situations that disturb your older one, where you simply illustrate what she is saying without any judgement or direction. This is an amazingly effective tool to help her work out her feelings. Don't feel the need to give the book a happy ending—leave it the way your child wants.

8. Read picture books about the arrival of a sibling and the sibling relationship. *Hello Baby!* by Lizzy Rockwell, The New Baby series by Rachel Fuller, *I Am a Big Brother* and *I Am a Big Sister* by Caroline Jayne Church, and *There Is a House Inside My Mummy* by Giles Andreae and Vanessa Cabban are powerful books about the transition to siblinghood. Books like *Spot's Baby Sister* by Eric Hill, *Albert and Little Henry* by Jez Alborough, *Tell Me What It's Like to be Big* by Joyce Dunbar and Debi Gliori, *Minty and Tink & No More Kissing* by Emma Chichester Clarke, and series like Blue Kangaroo by Emma Chichester Clarke and Alfie by Shirley Hughes provide vignettes of life with a sibling. You can start reading during the pregnancy itself,

continue after the baby arrives and read to the new baby herself as she grows older.

For more guidance on how to handle the sibling relationship, we highly recommend the book *Peaceful Parent, Happy Siblings* by Dr Laura Markham.

Box 15.3 Managing Twins: Tips from GBSI Admin Vidya Venkatesan

Sleep patterns of babies change with every regression, every milestone and for so many more reasons. Just when you feel a routine has been set, something new comes up and it all goes haywire. With twins, it just feels twice as hard.

Here are some of the things that worked for us and some of the things that did not:

1. Having realistic expectations about sleep is important with one child. With twins, it is easier to have a nervous breakdown, so keeping your expectations realistic about baby sleep and seeking help when needed is important.

2. Babywearing was probably what kept us sane until the twins turned at least 18 months old. We have tried every type of carrier there is. It helped us to hold the babies for naps during travel, sickness, teething and growth spurts.

3. Co-sleeping is a lifesaver. I would not have done it any other way. It is tough to find time to rest as a breastfeeding mother. With twins, if you are not nursing lying down, there is just no possibility of resting. If I had to wake up with each of them, pick them up from the cribs, nurse, wait until they fall asleep and place

them in the crib only to have to do it again, I would not have
continued breastfeeding them as long as I did.

4. Music/white noise helped us in the initial months to make sure
   one baby did not wake the other. Over time they learnt to sleep
   through each other's noise.

5. Having a bedtime routine is critical. At 4 months, we started a
   bedtime routine of bath, changing into pyjamas, dimming lights
   in their room and listening to some bedtime songs—which gave
   them the signal that it's bedtime.

6. Seeking additional help from your spouse, family, nanny is okay.
   Young babies need our help (by being present close to them) even
   when they sleep as they don't have the ability to soothe themselves
   to sleep yet. With two of them, it's hard holding them for naps.
   When they were young, we used to nap them in different rooms
   where I would lie down next to one of them and my nanny would
   watch the other twin. This way it is easy to catch them when they
   stir to pat/nurse them back to sleep.

7. Since there are two babies, it is also important to be flexible. What
   works with one baby may not necessarily work with the other.

16

The Magical Ritual of Bedtime Reading

There is one sleep aid and magical ritual that we have not yet touched upon. This is something very close to our hearts. It is reading picture books to our babies and children.

'Reading to our children? How is that connected to sleep?' you may ask. Unrelated though it may seem, any book-loving family knows that nothing nudges us off into dreamland as seamlessly as a good bedtime book. And while we know it works for an adult or a teenager, the fact is that it serves the same purpose absolutely beautifully for babies too.

Of course, babies will *not* nod off to sleep while being read to. Life is definitely not that simple! But sharing books is one of the most powerful components of any bedtime or pre-nap routine. Whether it is thumbing through touch and feel books with our infants or reading the same book numerous times to our toddler or entering the immersive universe of a book series with our pre-schooler, books are a wonderful signal to the child that it's time to unwind now. Reading acts as a bridge between fast-paced action and slowing down, between the world outside the bedroom and the land of dreams, between outer and inner worlds, between separation from the parent and connection with us. It makes the transition to sleep enjoyable, not something to be detested and resisted.

It is possible to read books to even the youngest of babies. In fact, both of us read to our children while they were still in the womb. We may have felt a bit silly as our husbands lovingly recited stories to our bellies, but we had learned that even unborn babies tune in to the rhythm and cadence of our voices. Parts of the brain that process language get stimulated. We read to our babies the first day we returned from the hospital as well. Newborns start to understand how words and sentences fit together as language networks are formed in their brains. They start developing cognition, forming mental pictures and connections. In fact, early reading by parents is intricately linked to later literacy skills. The sheer volume of words, the breadth of language, the rhythm and repetition and the association with pictures was something we could never replicate in mere conversation.

In fact, introducing babies to books has several benefits. They learn to value books and stories at a young age and can create the foundation for a lifelong love of reading. Picture books spark their imagination and stimulate their curiosity. Books help to foster social and communication skills. They help in the development of emotional empathy (the ability to experience the reactions to the observed experience of another) and also cognitive empathy or theory of mind (the ability to adapt to another's viewpoint). Books also help to develop 'joint attention', an important milestone where the child gains the ability to *share focus* with someone else, to observe the same thing as another person and know that it is a joint experience. The nuances of joint attention, like the child herself initiating it

('Look, papa, it's a fire truck!') or the child wanting the parent to acknowledge the shared experience ('Yes, that's right, it *is* a fire truck!') are facilitated beautifully by reading books together.

Reading with babies and toddlers also helps to build attention span and concentration. While listening to stories, they are rewarded for being focused, for paying attention and for remembering things because that is how the story progresses.

Books also widen a child's horizons and allow her to gain knowledge about places, people and things she has not encountered as yet—whether it is a zebra or a spaceship or a faraway culture. This provides a lot of background information with which to make sense of the world. Stories about events like starting school or a parent resuming work or the arrival of a new sibling help them to process these new experiences. Books can also be an effective alternative to screen time for toddlers.

For children to receive all of these magical gifts from reading, it is very important for reading to be a pleasurable activity. They should see their parents exhibit enthusiasm about the phenomenon. They should feel joy when they read. Their bodies should relax and fill with happy hormones. So, bedtime reading is actually the happy meeting point of both our desire to build a love for books in our babies and our need for a transition ritual into sleep. Cuddling up with a book releases oxytocin in both the baby and the parent. It is a loving, joyous experience. It is a time for bonding and for reconnecting after a long day. It creates happy associations with words and pictures on the page, while also filling our babies' cups and relaxing them for the final stage of soothing.

If you have been reading to your baby from Day 1, the relationship with books will likely grow organically. If you are thinking about how to introduce books to your little one, here are some ideas:

- Newborn babies are able to perceive black-and-white and high-contrast books. At the same time, you can also read to them from storybooks because hearing you relate a story is enjoyable for them as well. It's a good idea to use board books, flap books, sound books and touch-and-feel books for younger babies.

- Build a culture of reading by having lots of books in the house. Have some books in every room that the baby spends time in. Keep rotating the books that are available to the baby so that the baby encounters new and interesting material regularly.

- When placing the baby on the floor or on a bed to play with scattered toys, include two or three books in the assortment for the baby to explore. When engaging in pre-nap or bedtime reading, have a stack of books for the baby to sift through.

- Don't worry about finishing a book. Let the baby hop from book to book. Toddlers usually do listen to complete books, but, again, there is no hard and fast rule.

- Use lots of voices, sound effects, facial expressions and gestures when reading aloud from books.

- Feel free to change some words or the entire language to make it easier for the baby to understand.

- Feel free to read books in different languages. Bilingualism and multilingualism are good for baby brains!

- Point out interesting things in the illustrations that the baby can relate with.

- Don't focus on 'teaching' the baby anything. Let the baby enjoy the books.

- Follow your child's lead. If the baby wants to read a book six times, please oblige him!

- Figure out where to source books from. Most local bookshops do not have high-quality children's literature. Join a children's library, follow children's reading groups or influencers on social media, visit bookshops with dedicated children's book sections and knowledgeable store owners.

Bedtime reading has served our families beautifully and has been adopted by many parents we advise with great success and joy. Most parents count it to be one of the happiest points of their day. This is an investment well worth some time, money and effort. To get you started, we are happy to suggest some 'all-time hits' from our home libraries! We hope this will lead to some wonderful, cosy moments with your babies and set your children up for a lifetime of reading.

Box 16.1 Bedtime Reading Suggestions

While book suggestions are grouped by age, there is much overlap and most books easily work for a span of one year before and after that age as well, if not two years.

0–1 year

- *If You See a Kitten*; *Whose Baby Am I?*; *Who Says Woof?* —all by John Butler
- The Spot series by Eric Hill
- *What the Ladybird Heard* (sound book), *Toddle Waddle*, *The Gruffalo*—all by Julia Donaldson
- *A Beary Tale* by Anthony Browne

- *Where's My Teddy?*; *Six Little Chicks*; *Hug*—all by Jez Alborough
- *In the Tall Tall Grass*; *In the Small Small Pond*; *Barnyard Banter*—all by Denise Fleming
- *Dogs* by Emily Gravett
- *Dear Zoo*; *Oh Dear!*—by Rod Campbell
- *The Very Hungry Caterpillar*; *Brown Bear, Brown Bear, What Do You See?* by Eric Carle
- *Silly Suzy Goose*; *Look Out Suzy Goose*—by Petr Horacek
- *Tails*; *Heads*; *Dogs*—all by Matthew van Fleet
- *Goodnight Gorilla* by Peggy Rathman
- *Goodnight Moon* by Margaret Wise Brown
- *What Does Baby Want* by Tupera Tupera
- *Boo Boo Baby and The Giraffe* by Eileen Browne and Emily Bolam
- Books by Karen Katz
- *Dream Animals* by Emily Winfield

1–2 years

- *Elephantantrum* by Gillian Shields
- *Goat Goes to Playgroup*; *Chocolate Mousse for Greedy Goose*—by Julia Donaldson
- *Egg* by Kevin Henkes
- The Elmer series by David McKee
- Campbell push–pull–slide books
- *Truck, Truck, Goose* by Tammi Sauer
- The Gajapati Kulapati series by Ashok Rajagopalan
- *Little Blue Truck* by Alice Schertle
- *We're Going on a Bear Hunt* by Michael Rosen and Helen Oxenbury
- *Maisy Goes to Bed* by Lucy Cousins

- *Giraffes Can't Dance* by Giles Andreae
- *I Love You Night and Day* by Smriti Prasadam-Halls
- *Guess How Much I Love You* by Sam McBratney and Anita Jeram

2–3 years

- The Very Cranky Bear series by Nick Bland
- *The Tiger Who Came to Tea* by Judith Kerr
- *A House in the Woods* by Inga Moore
- *Kiss It Better* by Smriti Prasadam-Halls
- *Stormy* by Guojing
- How to Tuck in Your Sleepy Lion series by Jane Clarke
- Books by Julia Donaldson
- *A Brave Bear* by Sean Taylor and Emily Hughes
- *How to Catch a Star* by Oliver Jeffers
- *The Day the Crayons Quit* by Drew Daywalt and Oliver Jeffers
- *Pickle Mania* by Srividhya Venkat
- *The Rabbit Listened* by Cori Doerrfeld
- *The Koala Who Could* by Rachel Bright and Jim Field
- *A Sick Day for Amos McGee* by Philip C. Stead
- *Ammachi's Glasses* by Priya Kuriyan
- *Nani's Walk to the Park* by Deepa Balsavar
- *Florentine and Pig and the Spooky Forest Adventure* by Eva Katzler and Jess Mikhail
- *Bringing Down the Moon* by Jonathan Emmett and Vanessa Cabban
- *And Tango Makes Three* by Justin Richardson, Peter Parnell, Henry Cole

3–5 years

- *Oh the Places You'll Go!* by Dr Seuss
- *Eliza and the Moonchild* by Emma Chichester Clarke
- *Tidy* by Emily Gravett
- *A Walk in the Park* by Anthony Browne
- Series like Mog by Judith Kerr; Blue Kangaroo by Emma Chichester Clarke; Alfie by Shirley Hughes
- *Here We Are; What We'll Build*—by Oliver Jeffers
- *The Bear and the Piano* by David Litchfield
- *Lunchtime; The Something; Aunt Amelia*—all by Rebecca Cobb
- *If I Built A House* series by Chris van Dusen
- The Hairy MacLary series by Lynley Dodd
- *The Library Lion* by Michelle Knudsen and Kevin Hawkes
- *The Scariest Thing of All* by Debi Gliori
- *The Night Monster* by Sushree Mishra and Sanket Pethkar
- *Princess Easy Pleasy* by Natash Sharma and Priya Kuriyan
- *Vincent Can't Sleep* by Barb Rosenstock and Mary Grandpre

Acknowledgements

If it takes a village to raise a child, it certainly takes several to write a book. We're so grateful to have found a whole constellation of them to champion our book from the time it was barely a seed of an idea.

There would be no book without our three children—Sahir, Devika and Yamini—who popped into our world and took us on an incredible adventure. Along the way, they knocked down the grandest cliché of parenting—that parents know better than their children—because much of the wisdom we gathered came from them, and from learning to listen to their perfectly precise cues from the time they were born. Thanks to them for cracking open the magically meticulous nature of human sleep and protesting every time we took a wrong turn. We followed your cues and look where it got us!

Leading the support network Gentle Baby Sleep India on Facebook since 2016 connected us with a community of parents who, with their commitment to the art and science of baby-led sleep, nourished this project in their own way. To Dharini Bhaskar, our hat-tip for being a marvellously intuitive parent and a true wizard with words. Her endless kindness and that essential nudge to write this book meant the world. We are grateful to her for believing in this project vociferously, for being one of the first and most enthusiastic readers of the manuscript, for her observations, insights, experience and her wildly generous endorsement.

The hugest thanks to our Gentle Baby Sleep India village that served as the springboard for the book. To our volunteer team made up of extraordinary mums who have served as admins and peer counsellors over the years—you are the beating heart of our thriving group. To the thousands of parent members who stand up for their children through their sleep journey despite all the cultural and practical hurdles. To Himani Dhaundiyal, for being a solid sounding board from across many seas and her unparalleled humour that frequently lightened the load. Cheers to the other focus group mammas: Divya Chandrahas Mehta, Madhur Panjwani and Vidya Vijayan Sajith for reading the book closely, giving it space in their busy lives and sharing their thoughts on it. Mallika Ramaswamy, Rishika Vipin Menon, Sneha Jain Ashok, Vidya Venkatesan, Gurpriya Bagga, Ramneek Nitesh Gupta, Gurpreet Kaur and Nidhi Doshi, for sharing their personal stories of dealing with baby sleep with tenderness and parental instincts firmly in place.

To Professor James McKenna, for his overwhelming support and deeply enriching foreword and for going above and beyond to hold this book up high. His revolutionary work at the Mother–Baby Behavioral Sleep Laboratory inspired us to go with our instincts as parents; so, it's enormously gratifying to have him open the book. To Professor Helen Ball, Dr Tracy Cassels, Nupur Dhingra Paiva, Dr Anupam Sibal and Effath

Yasmin for reading the book with interest and endorsing it so warmly.

To Kanishka Gupta, for representing the book with gusto. To the team at Penguin Random House India: our editor Meru Gokhale for seeing the value of this book as a mum and a publisher, for her instant encouragement and giving it a warm home; to our copyeditor Binita Roy for so patiently seeing it through the finishing line; to Shreya Punj and the rest of the team for their enthusiasm over the book and treating it as their own baby.

And thank you, dear parents, for holding this book in your hands when there is so much else to do. We are all in this together, united by tremendous love for our children, for all children. On our most challenging days, when everything seemed to go off tune, a precious bunch of parenting books miraculously put things in perspective for us. They gave us a new lens through which to view the complex parent–baby connection and it all began to make so much sense. These books, listed under Further Reading, were like the best kind of intuitive friends and became our bedside companions, telling us what we needed to hear—to listen to our children. They spoke to our deepest fears and anxieties, offering the key to conscious and happy parenting. We hope this book can do the same for you.

Neha would like to thank

My parents, Joyita and Manan, for the precious scaffolding over the years and for being my most loyal readers and loudest cheerleaders. Thank you for being such thoughtful grandparents and having unflinching faith in how we decided to raise Sahir.

My husband, Suveen, for being the extraordinarily compassionate parent every child deserves. You raise the bar of modern-day parenting just by following your instincts and it's a marvel to watch what a natural you are at it. You make me a better parent. Thanks for quietly indulging my love for sleep and making sure I got more than my share even on the most difficult nights. For being an incredible partner, the most patient listener, the best critic and for pushing me to do this book.

My sister, Nishtha, for being a swell aunt and playing big sister, despite being the younger one, when I need it the most.

My Nani, Purabi, for her astonishing love for words and writing and for leaving them behind for Sahir and me. I wish she and my paternal grandmother Ba, Urmila, could have held this book in their hands. Losing them both at the time of writing this book has left an imprint on these pages and I miss them more than I can say.

My friends and journalism colleagues, for their keen interest and encouragement.

My co-author and dear friend, Himani Dalmia, for suggesting we do this book together, springing from our shared parenting philosophy and making it such a pleasure to write and share with the world.

Himani would like to thank

My husband, Akash, for being absolutely in sync with me about tuning into our instincts as parents, following our babies' leads and making our family front and centre of our lives; for teaching me much of what I now know about baby sleep with incredible observation and instinctual problem-solving skills;

for supporting me on what was a crazy passion project, before it became a vital cause and line of work.

My parents, Nilanjana and V.N. Dalmia, for being doting grandparents and always staying abreast of the 'new-fangled' ideas I would share (which were really not very different from their own ideals).

My brother, Pranav, for being a friend, a listener and an adoring uncle to his nieces, and for having my back in the practical world while I devoted myself to motherhood.

My mother-in-law, Bandana Sen, in whose eyes we saw a reflection of our own love for our daughters, who supported us every step of the way as we held, nursed, nurtured and followed our babies—we lost you too early, but the seeds of love you sowed in your granddaughters and the legacy of books and culture you left behind will last them a lifetime.

And finally, my friend and kindred spirit, Neha Bhatt, who reinforced my parenting beliefs at every step, was a shoulder to cry on after tough days and sleepless nights, and who showed me the way as I embarked on motherhood a year behind her. I could not have asked for a better co-parent for this book.

References

Foreword

H. Ball, C. Tomori, and James J. McKenna. 2020. 'Toward an integrated anthropology of infant sleep'. American Anthropologist 121 (3): 595–61.

P.S. Blair, H.L. Ball, J.J. McKenna, L. Feldman-Winter, K.A. Marinelli, M.C. Bartick, and Academy of Breastfeeding Medicine. (2020). 'Bedsharing and breastfeeding: The Academy of Breastfeeding medicine protocol #6, Revision 2019'. Breastfeeding Medicine 15 (1): 5–16. doi:10.1089/bfm.2019.29144.psb

Sean C.L. Deoni, Douglas C. Dean 3rd, Irene Piryatinsky, Jonathan O'Muircheartaigh, Nicole Waskiewicz, Katie Lehman, Michelle Han, and Holly Dirks. 2013. 'Breastfeeding and early white matter development: a cross sectional study'. Neuroimage 82: 77–86.

K. A. Marinelli, H.L. Ball, J.J. McKenna, and P.S. Blair. 2019. 'An integrated analysis of maternal infant sleep, breastfeeding, and sudden infant death syndrome research supporting a balance discourse'. Journal of Human Lactation 35 (3): 510–20. doi:10.1177/0890334419851797.

J.J. McKenna. 2018. 'Human mother–infant dyad'. In The International Encyclopedia of Biological Anthropology, edited by W. Trevathan, M. Cartmill, D. Dufour, C. Larsen, D. O'Rourke, K. Rosenberg and K.Strier. doi:10.1002/9781118584538.ieba0539.

James J. McKenna, Helen Ball, Lee T. Gettler. 2007. 'Mother–infant co-sleeping, breastfeeding and sudden infant death syndrome: What biological anthropology has discovered about normal infant sleep and pediatric sleep medicine'. Yearbook of Physical Anthropology 50:133–61.

J.J. McKenna and L.T. Gettler. 2016a. 'There is no such thing as infant sleep, there is not such thing as breastfeeding, there is only breastsleeping'. Acta Paediatrica 105: 17–21.

J.J. McKenna and L.T. Gettler. 2016b. 'Supporting a "bottom-up", no holds barred, psych-anthro-pediatrics: Making room (scientifically) for bedsharing families'. Sleep Medicine Reviews. doi:10.1016/j.smry.2016.06.003

Mercedes F. Paredes, David James, Sara Gil-Perotin, Hosung Kim, Jennifer A Cotter, Carissa Ng, Kadellyn Sandoval, David H Rowitch, Duan Xu, Patrick S McQuillen, Jose-Manuel Garcia-Verdugo, Eric J. Huang, Arturo Alvarez-Buylla. 2016. 'Extensive migration of young neurons into the infant human frontal lobe'. Science 354163081, doi: 10.1126/science.aaf7073 .

Chapter 1

American Academy of Pediatrics. n.d. 'Sleeping and Eating Issues'. https://www.aap.org/en-us/advocacy-and-policy/aap-health-initiatives/practicing-safety/Documents/Sleeping_Eating%20Issues.pdf.

Jen Christensen. 2017. 'Our Ancient Ancestors May Have Slept Better than You, but Less', CNN Health, 23 June. https://edition.cnn.com/2015/10/29/health/sleep-like-your-ancestors/index.html.

Michaeleen Doucleff. 2018. 'Is Sleeping with Your Baby as Dangerous as Doctors Say?' NPR, 21 May 2018. https://www.npr.org/

sections/goatsandsoda/2018/05/21/601289695/is-sleeping-with-your-baby-as-dangerous-as-doctors-say.

Carlos González. 2012. *Kiss Me*. London: Pinter & Martin.

Trisha Korioth. January 2013. 'Safe and Sound: Tips for Using Infant Swings'. AAP News. https://www.aappublications.org/content/34/1/25.5.

James J. McKenna and Lee T. Gettler. 2007. 'Mother-Infant Cosleeping with Breastfeeding in the Western Industrialized Context'. https://cosleeping.nd.edu/assets/29735/gettler_co_sleep.bio_cultural.pdf.

James J. McKenna and Edmund P. Joyce. 2008. 'Cosleeping and Biological Imperatives: Why Human Babies Do Not and Should Not Sleep Alone'. *Neuroanthropology*, 21 December 2008. https://neuroanthropology.net/2008/12/21/cosleeping-and-biological-imperatives-why-human-babies-do-not-and-should-not-sleep-alone/.

Jodi A. Mindell, Avi Sadeh, Benjamin Wiegand, Ti Hwei How, Daniel Y.T. Goh. 2010. 'Cross-Cultural Differences in Infant and Toddler Sleep'. *Sleep Medicine* 11 (3): 274–80. https://pubmed.ncbi.nlm.nih.gov/20138578/.

Darcia Narvaez. 2010. 'Research Shows Child Rearing Practices of Distant Ancestors Foster Morality, Compassion in Kids'. *Notre Dame News*, 17 September 2010. https://news.nd.edu/news/research-shows-child-rearing-practices-of-distant-ancestors-foster-morality-compassion-in-kids/.

Hannah Piosczyk, Nina Landmann, Johannes Holz, Bernd Feige, Dieter Riemann, Christoph Nissen and Ulrich Voderholzer. 2014. 'Prolonged Sleep under Stone Age Conditions'. *Journal of Clinical Sleep Medicine* 10 (7): 719–22. https://www.ncbi.nlm.nih.gov/pmc/articles/PMC4067433/.

Brooke Richardson. 2013. 'Exploring Mother-Infant Bedsharing Through a Cross-Cultural Lens: Western Versus Non-Western Mother-Infant Sleep Arrangements'. *Journal of the Motherhood Initiative* 4 (2): 120–29.

Sree Roy. 2018. 'Despite Bedsharing, Indian-Americans Have Fewer Sudden Infant Deaths'. *Sleep Review*, 10 September 2018. https://www.sleepreviewmag.com/sleep-health/demographics/race-ethnicity/despite-bedsharing-indian-americans-fewer-sudden-infant-deaths/.

Mina Shimizu, Heejung Park and Patricia M. Greenfield. 2014. 'Infant Sleeping Arrangements and Cultural Values among Contemporary Japanese Mothers'. *Frontiers in Psychology*, 19 August 2014. https://www.ncbi.nlm.nih.gov/pmc/articles/PMC4137277/.

Kate Wong. 2012. 'Why Humans Give Birth to Helpless Babies'. *Scientific American*, 28 August 2012. https://blogs.scientificamerican.com/observations/why-humans-give-birth-to-helpless-babies/.

Chapter 2

Center for Disease Control and Prevention. 2017. 'How Much Sleep Do I Need?'. https://www.cdc.gov/sleep/about_sleep/how_much_sleep.html.

David Foulkes. 1999. *Children's Dreaming and the Development of Consciousness*. Cambridge, MA: Harvard University Press. https://psycnet.apa.org/record/1999-02151-000.

Sleep Foundation. 2020. 'How Sleep Affects Immunity'. 19 November 2020. https://www.sleepfoundation.org/physical-health/how-sleep-affects-immunity.

Elaine K.H. Tham, Nora Schneider and Birit F.P. Broekman. 2017. 'Infant Sleep and Its Relation with Cognition and Growth'. *Nature and Science of Sleep*, 15 May 2017. https://www.ncbi.nlm.nih.gov/pmc/articles/PMC5440010/.

Tarja Porkka-Heiskanen and Anna V. Kalinchuk. 2010. 'Adenosine, Energy Metabolism and Sleep Homeostasis'. *Sleep Medical Review*, 20 October 2010. https://pubmed.ncbi.nlm.nih.gov/20970361/.

Matthew Walker. 2018. *Why We Sleep: The New Science of Sleep and Dreams*. London: Penguin Books.

The World Health Organization. 2019. 'To Grow Up Healthy, Children Need to Sit Less and Play More'. 24 April 2019. https://www.who.int/news/item/24-04-2019-to-grow-up-healthy-children-need-to-sit-less-and-play-more.

Chapter 3

Marc Weissbluth. 2014. *Healthy Sleep Habits, Happy Child*. New York: Random House.

S.E. Anderson, R. Andridge and R.C. Whitaker. 2016. 'Bedtime in Preschool-Aged Children and Risk for Adolescent Obesity'. *Journal of Pediatrics* 176: 17–22.

H.L. Ball. 2003. 'Breastfeeding, Bed-Sharing, and Infant Sleep'. *Birth* 30: 181–88. https://doi.org/10.1046/j.1523-536X.2003.00243.x.

H.L. Ball. 2006. 'Parent–Infant Bed-Sharing Behavior'. *Human Nature* 17 (3): 301–18. http://www.springerlink.com/index/0XVDFP8G88LW22AQ.pdf.

H.L. Ball, and P.K. Klingaman. 2007. 'Breastfeeding and Mother–Infant Sleep Proximity: Implications for Infant Care'. In *Evolutionary Medicine and Health: New Perspectives*. New York: Oxford University Press, pp. 226–41

C.E. Gribbin, S.E. Watamura, A. Cairns, J.R. Harsh and M.K. LeBourgeois. 2012. 'The Cortisol Awakening Response (CAR) in 2-to 4-Year-Old Children: Effects of Acute Nighttime Sleep Restriction, Wake Time, and Daytime Napping'. *Developmental Psychobiology* 54 (4): 412–22.

James McKenna and L.T. Gettler. 2007. 'Mother-Infant Cosleeping with Breastfeeding in the Western Industrialized Context'. In T. Hale and P. Hartmann, *Textbook of Human Lactation*. Hale Publishing, p. 3. https://cosleeping.nd.edu/assets/29735/gettler_co_sleep.bio_cultural.pdf.

James McKenna. 2007. *Sleeping with Your Baby: A Parent's Guide to Co-Sleeping*. Platypus Press.

James McKenna & L.T. Gettler. 2011. 'Evolutionary Perspectives on Mother–Infant Sleep Proximity and Breastfeeding in a Laboratory Setting'. *American Journal of Physical Anthropology* 144 (3): 454–62.

James McKenna and L.T. Gettler. 2016. 'There Is No Such Thing as Infant Sleep, There Is No Such Thing as Breastfeeding, There Is Only Breastsleeping'. *Acta Paediatrica* 105 (1): 17–21.

J.A. Mindell and A.A. Williamson. 2018. 'Benefits of a Bedtime Routine in Young Children: Sleep, Development, and Beyond'. *Sleep Medicine Review* 40: 93–108. https://www.ncbi.nlm.nih.gov/pmc/articles/PMC6587181/.

S. Mosko, C. Richard and James McKenna. 2007. 'Infant Arousals during Mother–Infant Bed Sharing: Implications for Infant Sleep and Sudden Infant Death Syndrome Research'. *Pediatrics* 100 (5): 841–49.

R.A. Schön and M. Silvén. 2007. 'Natural Parenting: Back to Basics in Infant Care'. *Evolutionary Psychology* 5 (1): 102–83.

Douglas M. Teti, Bo-Ram Kim, Gail Mayer, and Molly Countermine. 2007. 'Maternal Emotional Availability at Bedtime Predicts Infant Sleep Quality'. *Journal of Family Psychology* 24 (3): 307–15.

Chapter 4

Kimberly C. Starr. 2019. 'Scientific Evidence: Are Sleep Regressions Real?', Sleeptrainingkids.com, 19 August. https://sleeptrainingkids.com/scientific-evidence-are-sleep-regressions-real/.

Marc Weissbluth. 2014. *Healthy Sleep Habits, Happy Child*. New York: Random House.

Chapter 5

Alison Gopnik. 2017. *The Gardener and the Carpenter*. Penguin Random House.

Y. Harrison. 2004. 'The Relationship between Daytime Exposure to Light and Night-Time Sleep in 6–12-Week-Old Infants'. *Journal of Sleep Research* 13 (4): 345–52. https://onlinelibrary.wiley.com/doi/pdf/10.1111/j.1365-2869.2004.00435.x.

D. Joseph, N.W. Chong, M.E. Shanks, E. Rosato, N.A. Taub, S.A. Petersen and M. Wailoo. 2015. 'Getting Rhythm: How Do Babies Do It?', *Archives of Disease in Childhood-Fetal and Neonatal Edition* 100 (1): F50–F54. https://fn.bmj.com/content/fetalneonatal/100/1/F50.full.pdf.

S. Kitzinger. 1975. 'The Fourth Trimester?' *Midwife Health Visit Community Nurse* 11(4):118–21.

Chapter 6

American Academy of Pediatrics. N.d. 'Infant Food and Feeding'. https://www.aap.org/en-us/advocacy-and-policy/aap-health-initiatives/HALF-Implementation-Guide/Age-Specific-Content/Pages/Infant-Food-and-Feeding.aspx.

Australian Government, Department of Health. 2011. 'Breastfeeding'. https://www1.health.gov.au/internet/publications/publishing.nsf/Content/gug-carer-toc-gug-carer-breastfeeding.

Rowena Bennett. 2017. *Your Baby's Bottle-Feeding Aversion, Reasons and Solutions*. Ingram.

Michael A. Grandner, Nicholas Jackson, Jason R. Gerstner and Kristen L. Knutson. 2013. 'Dietary Nutrients Associated with Short and Long Sleep Duration: Data from a Nationally Representative Sample'. *Appetite* 64: 71–80. https://www.ncbi.nlm.nih.gov/pmc/articles/PMC3703747/.

Katri Peuhkuri, Nora Sihvola and Riitta Korpela. 2012. 'Diet Promotes Sleep Duration and Quality'. *Nutrition Research* 32 (5): 309–19.

UNICEF. N.d. 'Early Childhood Nutrition'. https://www.unicef.org/india/what-we-do/early-childhood-nutrition.

Noah Voreades, Anne Kozil and Tiffany L. Weir. 2014. 'Diet and
    the Development of the Human Intestinal Microbiome'.
    Frontiers in Microbiology 5: 494. https://www.frontiersin.org/
    articles/10.3389/fmicb.2014.00494/full.

E.J. Watson, S. Banks, A.M. Coates and M.J. Kohler. 2017. 'The
    Relationship Between Caffeine, Sleep, and Behavior in Children'.
    Journal of Clinical Sleep Medicine 13 (4): 533–43. https://doi.
    org/10.5664/jcsm.6536.

The World Health Organization. 2011. 'Exclusive Breastfeeding for
    Six Months Best for Babies Everywhere'. https://www.who.int/
    news/item/15-01-2011-exclusive-breastfeeding-for-six-months-
    best-for-babies-everywhere.

Yawen Zeng, Jiazhen Yang, Juan Du, Xiaoying Pu, Xiaomen Yang,
    Shuming Yang and Tao Yang. 2014. 'Strategies of Functional
    Foods Promote Sleep in Human Beings'. *Current Signal
    Transduction Therapy* 9 (3): 148–55. https://www.ncbi.nlm.nih.
    gov/pmc/articles/PMC4440346/.

Chapter 7

American Academy of Pediatrics. N.d. https://www.healthychildren.
    org/English/ages-stages/baby/feeding-nutrition/Pages/
    Discontinuing-the-Bottle.aspx.

Manisha Agarwal, S. Ghousia, Sapna Konde and Sunil Raj. 2012.
    'Breastfeeding: Nature's Safety Net'. *International Journal of
    Clinical Pediatric Dentistry* 5 (1): 49.

Gavin Bremner, Alan M. Slater and Scott P. Johnson. 2015. 'Perception
    of Object Persistence: The Origins of Object Permanence in
    Infancy'. *Child Development Perspectives* 9 (1): 7–13.

Camille W. Brune and Amanda L. Woodward. 2007. 'Social Cognition
    and Social Responsiveness in 10-Month-Old Infants'. *Journal of
    Cognition and Development* 8 (2): 133–58.

Katherine A. Dettwyler. 1995. 'A Time to Wean: The Hominid Blueprint for the Natural Age of Weaning in Modern Human Populations'. *Breastfeeding: Biocultural Perspectives*: 39–73.

Katherine A. Dettwyler. 1999. 'A Natural Age of Weaning'. Department of Anthropology, Texas A and M University. https://www.researchgate.net/publication/265185534_A_Natural_Age_of_Weaning. Systematic Review and Meta-Analysis'. *Acta Paediatrica* 104: 62–84.

Kathryn G. Dewey. 2001. 'Nutrition, Growth, and Complementary Feeding of the Brestfed Infant'. *Pediatric Clinics of North America* 48 (1): 87–104. https://www.sciencedirect.com/science/article/pii/S003139550570287X.

Richard G. Erskine. 2019. 'Child Development in Integrative Psychotherapy: Erik Erikson's First Three Stages.' *International Journal of Integrative Psychotherapy* 10: 11–34.

M. Keith Moore and Andrew N. Meltzoff. 1999. 'New Findings on Object Permanence: A Developmental Difference Between Two Types of Occlusion'. *British Journal of Developmental Psychology* 17 (4): 623–44.

S.M. Nainar and Shamsia Mohummed. 2004. 'Diet Counseling during the Infant Oral Health Visit'. *Pediatric Dentistry* 26 (5): 459–62.

F.C. Neiva, Débora Martins Cattoni, J.L. Ramos and Hugo Issler. 2003. 'Early Weaning: Implications to Oral Motor Development'. *Journal of Pediatrics* 79 (1): 7–12.

S. Scaglioni, C. Agostoni, R. De Notaris, G. Radaelli, N. Radice, M. Valenti, M. Giovannini and E. Riva. 'Early Macronutrient Intake and Overweight at Five Years of Age'. *International Journal of Obesity* 24 (6): 777–81.

Rachel Tham, Gayan Bowatte, Shyamali Chandrika Dharmage, Daniel J. Tan, Melisa X.Z. Lau, Xin Dai, Katrina J. Allen and

Caroline J. Lodge. 2015. 'Breastfeeding and the Risk of Dental Caries: A

Chapter 8

Kelly Mom. https://kellymom.com/category/ages/weaning/.
Kim John Payne. 2010. *Simplicity Parenting*, Ballantine Books.
SO-S Parenting. https://sarahockwell-smith.com/2014/08/10/how-to-gently-nightwean-a-breastfed-baby-or-toddler/.

Chapter 9

Thomas S. Dee and Hans Henrik Sievertsen. 2018. 'The Gift of Time? School Starting Age and Mental Health'. *Health Economics* 27: 781–802. https://doi.org/10.1002/hec.3638.
David Elkind. 2006. *The Power of Play*. Boston, MA: Da Capo Lifelong Books.
Alison Gopnik. 2017. *The Gardener and the Carpenter*. London: Picador.
Peter Gray. 2015. *Free to Learn*. New York: Basic Books.

Chapter 11

H. Isabella Lanza and Deborah A.G. Drabick. 2010. 'Family Routine Moderates the Relation between Child Impulsivity and Oppositional Defiant Disorder Symptoms'. Journal of Abnormal Child Psychology, 6 August. https://link.springer.com/article/10.1007/s10802-010-9447-5.

Chapter 12

The Australian Association for Infant Mental Health. November 2002, reviewed October 2013. https://www.aaimh.org.au/key-issues/position-statements-and-guidelines/AAIMHI-Position-paper-1-Controlled-crying.pdf.

Tracy Cassels. 'What You Need to Know about Crying-It-Out', Evolutionary Parenting. https://evolutionaryparenting.com/what-you-need-to-know-about-crying-it-out/.

Joan L. Luby, Deanna M. Barch, Andy Belden, Michael S. Gaffrey, Rebecca Tillman, Casey Babb, Tomoyuki Nishino, Hideo Suzuki and Kelly N. Botteron. 2012. 'Maternal Support in Early Childhood Predicts Larger Hippocampal Volumes at School Age'. National Academy of Sciences, 21 February. https://pubmed.ncbi.nlm.nih.gov/22308421/.

James J. McKenna and Edmund P. Joyce. 2008. 'Cosleeping and Biological Imperatives: Why Human Babies Do Not and Should Not Sleep Alone'. *Neuroanthropology*, 18 December.

Wendy Middlemiss, Douglas A. Granger, Wendy A. Goldberg and Laura Nathans. April 2012. 'Asynchrony of Mother-Infant Hypothalamic-Pituitary-Adrenal Axis Activity Following Extinction of Infant Crying Responses Induced during the Transition to Sleep'. *Early Human Development*. https://pubmed.ncbi.nlm.nih.gov/21945361/.

Sarah Ockwell Smith. 'Self Settling—What Really Happens When You Teach a Baby to Self Soothe to Sleep'. https://sarahockwell-smith.com/2014/06/30/self-settling-what-really-happens-when-you-teach-a-baby-to-self-soothe-to-sleep/.

Chapter 13

Eve R. Colson, Marian Willinger and Denis Rybin. 2013. 'Trends and Factors Associated with Bed-Sharing: The National Infant Sleep Position Study'. JAMA Pediatrics. https://www.ncbi.nlm.nih.gov/pmc/articles/PMC3903787/.

Michaeleen Doucleff. 2018. 'Is Sleeping with Your Baby as Dangerous as Doctors Say?' NPR, 21 May. https://www.npr.org/sections/

goatsandsoda/2018/05/21/601289695/is-sleeping-with-your-baby-as-dangerous-as-doctors-say.

Michael L. Macknin, Sharon VanderBrug Medendorp and Mary C. Maier. 1989. 'Infant Sleep and Bedtime Cereal', JAMA Pediatrics. https://jamanetwork.com/journals/jamapediatrics/article-abstract/514762.

Amy Mao, Melissa M. Burnham, Beth L. Goodlin-Jones, Erika E. Gaylor and Thomas F. Anders. 2004. 'A Comparison of the Sleep–Wake Patterns of Cosleeping and Solitary-Sleeping Infants'. Child Psychiatry and Human Development. https://link.springer.com/article/10.1007/s10578-004-1879-0.

Chapter 14

B. Adhisivam. 2012. 'Is Gripe Water Baby-Friendly?' Journal of Pharmacology and Pharmacotherapeutics. https://www.ncbi.nlm.nih.gov/pmc/articles/PMC3356971/.

Gwen Dewar. 'Finding the Right Infant Sleep Aid: 13 Evidence-Based Tips for Getting Your Baby to Sleep'. https://www.parentingscience.com/infant-sleep-aid.html.

'Effects of Pacifiers on Early Oral Development', International Journal of Orthodontics. https://europepmc.org/article/med/17256438?fbclid=IwAR1hhYwzNpIoyOj2xD0SQQ79lQrjeKj2IC0i_lfhxLa9CJk9RcD10bD2o64.

Anat Cohen Engler, Amir Hadash, Naim Shehadeh and Giora Pillar. 2012. 'Breastfeeding May Improve Nocturnal Sleep and Reduce Infantile Colic: Potential Role of Breast Milk Melatonin'. European Journal of Pediatrics. https://pubmed.ncbi.nlm.nih.gov/22205210/.

Dana Festila, Mircea Ghergie, Alexandrina Muntean, Daiana Matiz and Alin Serbanescu. 2014. 'Suckling and Non-Nutritive Sucking Habit: What Should We Know?' Clujul Medical, 30 January 30. https://www.ncbi.nlm.nih.gov/pmc/articles/PMC4462418/.

Marjo Niemelä, Outi Pihakari, Tytti Pokka, Marja Uhari and Matti Uhari. 2000. 'Pacifier as a Risk Factor for Acute Otitis Media: A Randomized, Controlled Trial of Parental Counseling'. Pediatrics. https://doi.org/10.1542/peds.106.3.483.

Chapter 15

B.M.F. Galdikas and J.W. Wood. 1990. 'Birth Spacing Patterns in Humans and Apes'. American Journal of Physical Anthropology 83 (2): 185–91. https://doi.org/10.1002/ajpa.1330830207.

Laura Markham. 2015. Peaceful Parent, Happy Siblings. TarcherPerigee.

Melissa Thompson. 2013. 'Comparative Reproductive Energetics of Human and Nonhuman Primates'. Annual Review of Anthropology 42: 287–304. https://www.researchgate.net/publication/274471909_Comparative_Reproductive_Energetics_of_Human_and_Nonhuman_Primates.

World Health Organization. Guidelines on screentime. https://apps.who.int/iris/bitstream/handle/10665/311664/9789241550536-eng.pdf?sequence=1&isAllowed=y.

Chapter 16

Scott J. Brown, Kyung E. Rhee and Sheila Gahagan. 2016. 'Reading at Bedtime Associated with Longer Nighttime Sleep in Latino Preschoolers'. Clinical Pediatrics 55 (6): 525–31. https://escholarship.org/content/qt3h93h92c/qt3h93h92c.pdf.

Angela D. Friederici, Noam Chomsky, Robert C. Berwick, Andrea Moro and Johan J. Bolhuis. 2017. 'Language, Mind and Brain'. Nature Human Behaviour 1 (10): 713–22. https://drive.google.com/file/d/1BJW_folpvqOxfCvsoTzsTYGlk2gaPy26/view.

Allison Gabouer and Heather Bortfeld. 2021. 'Revisiting How We Operationalize Joint Attention'. Infant Behavior and

Development 63: 101566. https://www.ncbi.nlm.nih.gov/pmc/articles/PMC8172475/.

Linda Gillespie. 2019. 'Reading with Babies Matters!' YC Young Children 74 (3): 86–88. https://openlab.bmcc.cuny.edu/ece-209-lecture-fall-2019-longley/wp-content/uploads/sites/77/2020/02/Gillespie-2019.pdf.

Susan L. Hall and Louisa C. Moats. 2014. 'Why Reading to Children Is Important'. Preface: Knowledge for Literacy: 22, https://www.shankerinstitute.org/sites/default/files/TEACH%20--LiteracyLadders2015_low.pdf#page=22.

K.K. Jasińska and L.A. Petitto. 2014. 'Development of Neural Systems for Reading in the Monolingual and Bilingual Brain: New Insights from Functional Near Infrared Spectroscopy Neuroimaging'. Developmental Neuropsychology 39 (6): 421–39. https://www.researchgate.net/profile/Kaja-Jasinska/publication/264939434_Development_of_Neural_Systems_for_Reading_in_the_Monolingual_and_Bilingual_Brain_New_Insights_From_Functional_Near_Infrared_Spectroscopy_Neuroimaging/links/5638b52508ae51ccb3cc9395/Development-of-Neural-Systems-for-Reading-in-the-Monolingual-and-Bilingual-Brain-New-Insights-From-Functional-Near-Infrared-Spectroscopy-Neuroimaging.pdf.

Susan H. Landry, Karen E. Smith, Paul R. Swank, Tricia Zucker, April D. Crawford and Emily F. Solari. 2012. 'The Effects of a Responsive Parenting Intervention on Parent–Child Interactions during Shared Book Reading'. Developmental Psychology 48 (4): 969. https://www.researchgate.net/profile/Paul-Swank/publication/51831766_The_Effects_of_a_Responsive_Parenting_Intervention_on_Parent-Child_Interactions_During_Shared_Book_Reading/links/0912f5097cf5ddf41c000000/The-Effects-of-a-Responsive-Parenting-Intervention-on-Parent-Child-Interactions-During-Shared-Book-Reading.pdf.

Janice Lariviere and Janet E. Rennick. 2011. 'Parent Picture-Book Reading to Infants in the Neonatal Intensive Care Unit as an

Intervention Supporting Parent-Infant Interaction and Later Book Reading.' Journal of Developmental and Behavioral Pediatrics 32 (2): 146–52. https://journals.lww.com/jrnldbp/Abstract/2011/02000/Parent_Picture_Book_Reading_to_Infants_in_the.11.aspx.

Janet L. Towell, Lydia Bartram, Susan Morrow and Susannah L. Brown. 2019. 'Reading to Babies: Exploring the Beginnings of Literacy'. Journal of Early Childhood Literacy. https://www.researchgate.net/profile/Lydia-Bartram/publication/332967998_Reading_to_babies_Exploring_the_beginnings_of_literacy/links/5df2a1454585159aa4792eb7/Reading-to-babies-Exploring-the-beginnings-of-literacy.pdf.

Further Reading

Lawrence J. Cohen. 2002. *Playful Parenting: An Exciting New Approach to Raising Children That Will Help You Nurture Close Connections, Solve Behavior Problems, and Encourage Confidence.* Ballantine Books, reprint edition.

Joanna Faber and Julie King. 2017. *How to Talk So Little Kids Will Listen: A Survival Guide to Life with Children Ages 2-7.* Piccadilly Press.

Carlos Gonzalez. 2020. *Kiss Me: How to Raise your Children with Love.* Pinter & Martin, 2nd edition.

Carlos Gonzalez. 2020. *My Child Won't Eat: How to Enjoy Mealtimes Without Worry.* YogaWords, 2nd edition.

Alison Gopnik. 2016. *The Gardener and the Carpenter: What the New Science of Child Development Tells Us about the Relationship between Parents and Children.* Farrar, Straus and Giroux.

Alfie Kohn. 2006. *Unconditional Parenting: Moving from Rewards and Punishments to Love and Reason.* Atria Books, 1st edition.

Jean Liedloff. 1989. *The Continuum Concept.* Penguin.

Laura Markham. 2012. *Peaceful Parent, Happy Kids.* TarcherPerigee.

Laura Markham. 2015. *Peaceful Parent, Happy Siblings.* TarcherPerigee.

James J. McKenna, 2020. *Safe Infant Sleep: Expert Answers to Your Cosleeping Questions.* Platypus Media, illustrated edition.

Gordon Neufeld and Gabor Maté. 2006. *Hold On to Your Kids: Why Parents Need to Matter More Than Peers*. Ballantine Books, reprint edition.

Sarah Ockwell-Smith. 2017. *The Gentle Discipline Book*. Piatkus.

Nupur Dhingra Paiva. 2017. *Love and Rage: The Inner Worlds of Children*. Yoda Press.

Kim John Payne. 2010. *Simplicity Parenting: Using the Extraordinary Power of Less to Raise Calmer, Happier, and More Secure Kids*. Ballantine Books.

Kim John Payne. 2015. *The Soul of Discipline: The Simplicity Parenting Approach to Warm, Firm, and Calm Guidance—From Toddlers to Teens*. Ballantine Books.

Daniel Siegel and Tina Payne Bryson. 2012. *The Whole-Brain Child: 12 Proven Strategies to Nurture Your Child's Developing Mind*. Constable & Robinson.

Diana West. 2010. *The Womanly Art of Breastfeeding: Completely Revised and Updated 8th Edition* (La Leche League International Book). Ballantine Books.

Index